T0006791

BABBLE ON

ANDREW BROBYN

BABBLE ON

A DRUG MEMOIR

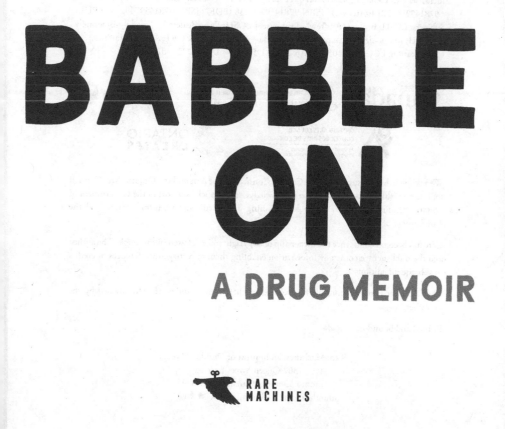

RARE MACHINES

Copyright © Andrew Brobyn, 2022

All rights reserved. No part of this publication may be reproduced, stored in a retrieval system, or transmitted in any form or by any means, electronic, mechanical, photocopying, recording, or otherwise (except for brief passages for purpose of review) without the prior permission of Dundurn Press. Permission to photocopy should be requested from Access Copyright.

Publisher: Scott Fraser | Acquiring editor: Julie Mannell
Cover designer: Laura Boyle
Cover image: shutterstock.com/Primsky

Library and Archives Canada Cataloguing in Publication

Title: Babble on : a drug memoir / Andrew Brobyn.
Names: Brobyn, Andrew, author.
Identifiers: Canadiana (print) 2022021252X | Canadiana (ebook) 20220212554 | ISBN 9781459749221 (softcover) | ISBN 9781459749238 (PDF) | ISBN 9781459749245 (EPUB)
Subjects: LCSH: Brobyn, Andrew—Drug use. | LCSH: Drug dealers—Canada—Biography. | LCSH: Manic-depressive persons—Canada—Biography. | LCGFT: Autobiographies.
Classification: LCC HV5805.B74 A3 2022 | DDC 364.1/3365092—dc23

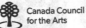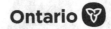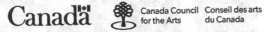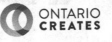

We acknowledge the support of the Canada Council for the Arts and the Ontario Arts Council for our publishing program. We also acknowledge the financial support of the Government of Ontario, through the Ontario Book Publishing Tax Credit and Ontario Creates, and the Government of Canada.

Care has been taken to trace the ownership of copyright material used in this book. The author and the publisher welcome any information enabling them to rectify any references or credits in subsequent editions.

The publisher is not responsible for websites or their content unless they are owned by the publisher.

Printed and bound in Canada.

Rare Machines, an imprint of Dundurn Press
1382 Queen Street East
Toronto, Ontario, Canada M4L 1C9
dundurn.com, @dundurnpress ⟨y⟩ f ⟨o⟩

Dedicated to those who get it.

Based on a true story, or something.

ONE
2012

Wait a tick.

Tick.

Why can I taste the acid?

Tick.

And why does it have a grainy texture?

Tick.

I loosen what feels like a mote of sand from one of the tabs and bite down. It bursts. My mouth is awash in a flavour I'd describe as grapefruit seeds of chemical regret, and I feel an instant coolness in my extremities. That's not good. This isn't good. I've heard stories, and done a lot of acid in my day, and seen a lot of fucked-up shit and bad trips, and the saying is "If it's bitter, it's a spitter." Also to be a burstable grain, that crystal must've been at least a milligram ... and some compounds are effective at doses in the microgram range. Most of that would've just absorbed into my mouth tissue immediately. *Tick.*

I follow the wisdom of countless mindless hippies before me and purge the tabs. I scrape my tongue for good measure. I can still taste the unique residue of impending psychosis, though, and start doing mental math in a futile race against my metabolism.

What sorts of compounds could one feasibly fit a full trip's worth of onto blotter paper? Which ones would taste like a crushed Tylenol daiquiri? How many micrograms, across five tabs, may have dissolved through my mucous membranes in the moments it's taken me to realize I've just dosed myself with a pretty hefty amount of a substance that I, and possibly even the manufacturer of said drug, have never tried before. Fuck.

There are too many options. In a split second, I curse every blessing I've ever made of all the renegade biochemists who've fuelled my lifelong quest to experience novel states of mental being. Fuck Hofmann. Fuck Shulgin. Fuck Nichols. This could be anything; all sorts of horrible medieval visions of Hell have been synthesized already, and more are being discovered in clandestine labs across the globe every day: DOB, 5-MeO-aMT, Bromo-DragonFLY, some sort of Aleph compound, 25I-NBOMe, 3-Quinuclidinyl benzilate ... the list is limitless (metaphorically, though verging on literally). My heartbeat picks up a semi-step and the contours sharpen around objects I hadn't even noticed I'm sharing this room with. The mind can be a prison, prism, and/or a palace; it's all about perception. I remind myself of the lessons of loony Tim Leary's take on *The Tibetan Book of the Dead*, and the (comparatively) more dependable Terence McKenna's *Food of the Gods*: set and setting are everything; your thoughts and physical presence must both reside in a safe space for the duration of the trip, unless you want to come out of it all animal — a devolved, semi-reptilian monstrosity wearing your epidermis: a silicone suit on an animated, proto-mammalian mannequin. I focus my attentions to mindfulness tactics and search my body for sensation ...

Yeah, *something's* off all right. Usually my psychedelic-state synesthesia isn't this all-encompassing. Did I just chew off a piece of the fucking Loc-Nar?

Is this the drug, or the predrug placebo? Either way, the paranoia's persistent, but considering that I, very stupidly, *took* five tabs from the untested sheet all at once, I'll go ahead and assume this is just the normal, ambient level of anxiety that I should naturally be feeling. I'm already about ten minutes down, anyway, so at least I know I'm not allergic to this — otherwise my heart wouldn't be palpitating quite so much as just permanently on pause. The real deal, once my mind makes it there, will be considerably more omnipersistent than a simple passing perception that I'm being watched, or that my watching is being sensed, or that the walls are breathing.

Should I go to the hospital? Call 911? No. I can't. I can feel the heat just thinking about it. No, this one's on me.

Maybe it was more like fifteen minutes, actually. Twenty? Time is all around me — the wall, my right wrist, the DVD player, my pocket — but it's all too far away to be any more than a blur, an oasis mirage in an ocean, a fading, disconcertingly coloured sunset.

Hmm. Maybe I should sit down. Better yet — lie down. That's the ticket. Also maybe this wasn't the best movie choice.

Apocalypse Now and LSD (ideally, properly synthesized LSD-25 — not that 1-propionyl-LSD or some other analogue bullshit): great combination. *Apocalypse Now* (*Redux*, I might add) and questionable amounts of an unknown research chemical: possibly less great. It might even be fair to classify this as *definitely* less great.

It's OK.

It's OK.

It's OK to have such a simple mantra in scenarios like this. *It's OK.* I've been in hairier situations before — I mean, obviously not like doing a gap-year tour in Vietnam, an M-16 graduation present courtesy of Uncle Sam, being experimented on with Agent Orange and a *Jacob's Ladder*, BZ-style, stimudeliriant — but drug-wise.

The thing about psychedelics (which I'm assuming I just cavalierly took some radical new sort of) is that they reveal that reality is subjective — even at the best of times — and it's kind of like a conversation taking place in many different languages at once. But this subjectivity is open to interpretation, and the drug is kind of like an interpreter: you get a good drug, you have a good conversation; you hit a bad tab, that conversation becomes a cacophony of sense overlaid with sense and stirred up until it's all nonsense.

I should probably turn off the movie now, but I really like this song, "The End." What a brilliant way to start a movie.

Tick.

What I really need now is a pad of paper, dim lighting, and a pack of crayons. The more colours, the better. Also I should probably put my knife down, somewhere out of immediate reach.

Tick.

Another thing I forgot about flicks a light on in the kitchen. My ex is standing in the doorway, metaphorically as always, but also actually, and clearly waiting for me to notice.

"It's four in the morning."

Tick.

That's a statement. I know she expects a response, but I've become somewhat less than the perfect suitor since our relationship started crumbling over the winter. We still live together, out of necessity, but that's changing in the next few days. I'm getting out of Dodge. I'm taking Java, my doggie — the *true* love of my life, and the only creature remotely capable of keeping me together — back *home*. Part border collie, part retriever, she acts like a coyote — playful, inquisitive, creative, sensitive, trusting ... with trust in me. She's my girl. I get Java; she's been mine since grade six, and she's mine now. My ex can keep the rest of our menagerie of pets: two cats, two ferrets, a rat, a snake, a few lizards ... a shitload of crickets. I'm cutting my losses.

My graduation ceremony was in January, and it was a shitshow. I didn't want to go. I knew what the end of my school career meant: no more easy ride, no more getting paid to show up at parties, no more learning what I wanted to and acing exams with the aid of the same grey-market nootropics I supply the professors and grad students with. My immediate plans are to liquidate my illicit assets, sell my client list, pack up shop, and retire to my parental home in the big city while I plan out what to do with a bachelor's degree in philosophy and about a quarter million in cash. It's not the end of the world, but no more psychedelic escapades at four in the morning for the conceivable future. I choose to leave her remark hanging there, choking on its obviousness.

"Can you, like, I don't know, turn it down? Or, like, go to sleep? Or whatever it is that *you* want to do, as long as it doesn't bother me? I have a job, remember? I have to, like, go to school in the morning."

Tick.

She's still waiting for me to say something. Or maybe she isn't — just letting her words permeate what she probably (rightly) assumes to be my drug-addled mind. I don't have anything to say. Not that I don't, generally. I have a Dead Sea's worth of salty things I'd like to share with her, but circumstance, brain chemistry, and a multiplicity of deep-seated personality flaws are preventing me from verbalizing my complicated feelings toward her.

Tick.

I don't have long to get rid of her before this becomes an all-out fiasco. Whatever it is that's coursing through my system is warping and contorting Colonel Kurtz's warbled "snail on a straight razor" tape-recorder monologue. I feel a keen sense of identity in kinship with the gastropod and its mystic spiral shell.

"So you're not even talking to me?"

Tick.

This is steadily getting worse. I really didn't want a fight. Especially not while I'm ostensibly engaged in research for *PiHKAL: The Next Frontier.* I feel a primeval Promethean energy stirring in my stomach, singeing butterfly cocoons shut. I need to defuse the situation, somehow assuage her skull-fucked sense of trust in me. I haven't been good at that lately, but I have to try — otherwise I'm in for six, to forty-eight, to an infinite expanse of hours full of excruciatingly introspective self-admonishment for every ill deed I've ever conceived — maybe a spot of formication. They call them *bad trips* for a reason.

—I love you. I love you so much. I'm sorry. I'm so sorry.

Tick.

Now she's speechless. Just like I should've remained. I sound like Stephen Hawking's animatronic voice saying something discomforting to his dog before its euthanasia. An increment of time passes that is somehow both relievingly short and unconsolingly long. A lemniscate of escape, before:

"No, you don't. You don't even love yourself. You don't even know what you're apologizing for anymore. I'm tired and going to bed. Good night."

She follows through on her threat and heads up to bed, leaving the light on in the kitchen. She knows I like being in the dark when I feel like shit.

Tick.

Oh, right. I forgot that I'm full on tripping, or — I hope this is the extent of the trip. Putting the ex situation out of mind for a second, I take a moment to assess my psychological state ...

Shit. Through the litany of pills and powders and syrups and smokes of all different sorts that I've consumed over the course of the last few days (my retirement party), I can't even distinguish just which discrepancies from reality are new to me. For all intents and purposes, everything is fucked.

Tick. Tick. Tick.

A sunrise spilling shadows from the TV-room windowsill sets a precedent for a sense of time that's elapsed while I've been — totally blanked out. Well, I suppose no recollection at all is likely better than whatever my subconscious self just experienced or endured.

Somehow I make the connection that dawn correlates to six or seven in the morning.

"You need to go. You need to get out." She's back and on the warpath, ready to attack in self-defence, if it comes to that.
Tick.
My time's up. If only this could be fixed by words.

In the Course of a Song

we'd listen to Chopin
spring waltz, nocturnes; nothing obscure

running through dreams, memories, plans
time and possibility

breathing, pressing
repeat ad infinitum

reducio ad absurdum
clucking, cooing, gobbledegooking

swelling up and pouring out
we filled an ocean with loss

we couldn't stop
we were so young

so strong
so perfect and right

for each other
and ourselves

it was poetry we never got
the chance to write;

why write when you can
live, there's nothing more

pure, or chaste
than living
for what we waste

A Bit of Context

This book was written over the course of around ten years. Some of that time, I was still involved in the illicit drug trade; much of that time, I was using an assortment of the various chemicals I'll be getting into more detail about later on; and for long periods, I have not been well, in a psychiatric sense. As a result, I've employed creative non-fiction to obscure the demarcations between what *really* happened, and what you are reading into a new reality. I don't remember everything exactly: identities have been warped, elements of some stories have been integrated into others, certain scenarios have been exaggerated, and others have been minimized. Think of this as a rap saga, or something. This is my legend.

As I said, for much of the time that I was writing, I was sick. This influenced how I wrote and also what I was afraid of saying and what I was uncompromising about saying. I am more forthcoming in this collection of stories than I would be in an interview. I often feel like a combination of a six-year-old and a centenarian: wise in my childishness and curious in my logic. As a result, my varied forms of artistic expression can come across as ... er ... confusion. But rest assured, while I may be confusing, I am also confused.

Sometimes I think of writing as a disease, almost as much a malediction as any of my actual diagnoses. It forces you to reimagine a scenario over and over, from a multitude of angles and opinions, and try to perfect it. You can't give up. You can't eat or sleep until it's done and written. Out of mind, out of sight. Like a good Baggie of yayo.

You'll probably notice that the timeline and tenses in this book are all fucked up and can be a little disorienting. This was not intentional. My memory isn't exactly functional at the best of times, and the ten years it took to write this book were not the best of times. I've done the best I can to help it seem to make sense, but I'm not a magician: I can't grant a wish or undo a spell of madness, much as I wish I could. Try to think of it as artistic or literary or creative or whatever you like. It might be more palatable that way.

[Set & Setting]
2012

Goose pimples.

Who makes that connection? Who spends their time ruminating on the relationship between the skins of some plucked poultry and these things blooming all over my body in epidermal effervescence? It doesn't even make sense. Pfft, pimples. Can you pop 'em? What about those bumps around your nipples? This broad I used to know said she got goop to come out of one, once. Probably lying, though. They're glands, aren't they? Those don't have goop in them — I think. I'll look it up later — I'll look her up, too. Fuck, forget it, way off track; I'm covered in these wannabe pimples or nipples, and I don't really give a nun's clit what they're all about. I just want this done. This is the worst part of my job, the waiting. I'm a punctual person, and that's pretty rare in this profession. So I end up waiting. A lot.

—Um, what's the time?

It's on the dash.

"Quarter past."

Shit. How is he so chill? Maybe that's not the right word. More like composed, or tranquilized. Damn near comatose.

I'm the chilled one. I should've anticipated the wait and worn more than this home-knit sweater. Or better yet, just told Grandma to get her shit together and knit a thicker, less itchy article of clothing. This is Canada. What in the hell was she thinking?

—Dude, he's late. Again.

My partner, Chud, grunts. Guess I'll have to go on that for now. I bow my head and scour the rubber mat under my feet for a flash of salvation — like some new age, post-relative morality, existential prostration: a perverse form of prayer, not that they aren't all warped and distorted ways of wishing upon some long since extinguished star. *Oh Sin, deliver me from god.* I use a lowercase *g* because, while I might believe in one, I don't respect it. I'm rewarded for tipping my cap to the fallen angels with a bent, slightly torn cigarette: this can work if I pinch it just so. I'm craving something stronger, but that would be a bad move at the moment.

—We look pretty bait ... Maybe we should take a trip around the block, or something.

"Sure."

He looks around, streetlights bouncing off his baldness, which he embraces with gumption, as he does all of life, by shaving any vestiges of hair he has left. We're sitting in his latest model Mercedes. His signature Danier black leather jacket, chain, and prescription designer nighttime shades make him seem like a Caucasian DMX. Versace socks and Gucci banana hammock. Ostentatious is an understatement. He's got a Mediterranean look about him, though, like he'd fit right in on a 150-foot private yacht in Beaulieu-sur-Mer. He comes across like a Sardinian human trafficker, evil, but laid back about it. He's probably less politically correct than either DMX or the human trafficker, though. He's fascinated by Putin — not, like, his personal views, but more about how he plays the game: how he moves the pieces, plucks the strings, strokes the brush. How he can make something happen with his words alone. He says everyone needs aspirations.

Under the jacket and Armani shirt, he has black tattoos up one arm with drops of purple, green, blue, and red dye dropped into the ink. They shine with iridescence. They're there to cover up an earlier tattoo he got out of a magazine, that barbed wire one every other kid who had a bone to pick with authority had gotten. He's common. He's a gold-standard hustler, even if he needs some liner notes about how not to look shady as a shit stain.

The engine sputters to life from its slip into hypothermic oblivion. The ghost in the machine is just as worn out and frigid as I am. It's early March, and we're in Canada … Did I mention that yet? Well, it bears repeating because it's cold here. Like, capital *C* Cold. The maybe/maybe-not goop-filled bumps on my nipples are harder than debating autonomous agency vs. material determinism with a plebeian vegetable case on life support.

They said I'd eventually get used to this weather when I got here from a magical place between the coasts of England and France, the Isle of Jersey. I didn't. Been here thirteen years now, and it's still as wretched as ever. Shitty thing is, I've lost my once-upon-a-time, so-called adorable accent and picked up most of the colloquialisms of this country (except that I still use words such as *wretched*, and *such as* rather than *like*, and *rather* instead of *instead of*), so I don't even have an excuse for not snowboarding, or liking hockey, or whatever. I fucking hate snow — magical my ass. Sure, at first when it's falling, it's all glittery, sparkling, pastel-like pixels, not so much white as every hue in the spectrum coalesced into one, the saturation jacked like it was on steroids — no shading. So I guess it has its infinitesimally momentous, momentary, aesthetic appeal — it's born beautiful. Congratulations, snow. But how many of these unique specks do we actually see as singular? How many individual flakes do we fully appreciate before they're crunch-consolidated into the tapestry under our tires? I don't think I can recall any particular piece of snow, just the broader concept of it.

People here just assume I'm Canadian, too, which I guess I am — but not Canadian like them. It's supposed to be a melting pot, right? But I think the burner under my part of the stove is defective. I'm always either frozen solid, or boiling over, never temperate, never bubbling away happily with the rest of the bland, pastiche, smorgasbord of a soup they conceitedly call their cultural collage.

I absent-mindedly pick at a scab on my arm as we hit the curb and take a right, merging with traffic. Public areas are the best option for these sorts of encounters. They ensure a mutual level of safety, or at least a mutually assured destruction. This element of comfort doesn't detract from the fact that I'm packing a jackknife in my pocket and have a straight razor tucked into my boot. My partner has the real ammunition (bear mace, taser, and — I'm not shitting you — a katana across the back seat). I'm more of a physical presence, though, which usually puts me in front.

My fingers quiver — it isn't a shiver due to the cold, more like a twitchy case of the jitters. They shouldn't, not after the forty milligrams of oxy up my nose. Granted, there's also half a gram of the only snow I can stand in there, keeping the

opiates company and shoving me down the well-lubed Slip 'N
Slide tube of coke-psychosis into a surrealistic, super-spatial,
super-sensory, synesthetic soliloquy of solipsistic, symbolism-
questioning semantics. Not to mention the two smiley-face
tabs gradually decomposing under my tongue, sabotaging any
semblance of sanity I could cling to in this sinking ship of a
"soul" I'm captaining. Still, I can't shake the feeling that something's about to go gravely awry. Of course, that could just be
paranoia, which is entirely understandable given the concen-
tration of illegal, alien alkaloids coursing through my nervous
system.

"I think I see him. It's go time, bud."

Nod in agreement. If I open my mouth, it might spew puke.

"Rippers after this?"

I grant another silent inclination of my mind (or, at least,
my head). He knows I get anxious before these meetings. An
unspoken bond exists between us. I turn off my personal phone
and my small-business phone. Then I check another phone: I
only use it once a week, but no messages. That's a relief; this
guy's impatient, despite the fact he's always late.

"It's gonna be fun, bro, amateur night."

—Mhmm.

We pull back through the parking lot and drive to a spot
equidistant between the two functioning lamps. The only
luminescent beams I perceive, though, are coming from phos-
phene dreams illuminating the illustrations on the insides of my
eyelids. He's waiting for us. We pop the trunk in anticipation
before getting out and walking the ten paces to a little, rusted
out, two-door, four-seat, shitbox sedan. I recognize the little
Slavic guy in the passenger seat, "Soulless," but not the big,
pockmarked guy driving. No matter, it's the little guy I care

about. He's tiny. Thin and short, rat-faced, near-eyes — all pupils … if he has irises, they're black. He's pale, with a few freckles and shaved-close black hair. Kid can't even grow a beard yet. I can hear Biggie Smalls's "Ten Crack Commandments" sung through fissures in the car's frame and briefly imagine laughing at what I think is perfect irony. I don't trust these guys to get the joke, though. The semi-tinted window rolls down. It's not even electric. Soulless speaks:

"Yo, sup. Your shit's in the trunk. On the left."

Chud (so named for several reasons), passes him a computer case jammed with $46,950 in multicoloured pieces of plasticky Monopoly-esque paper, and I pick up one of the three hockey bags from the trunk, careful not to slam the door down when closing it. He cares about that, for some reason — obviously not the noise, as Biggie pointedly reminds us all of rule number ten: something about *consignment*.

Chud and I nod at each other, nearly imperceptibly, and then at him. Following this practised, ersatz kowtow, I drop the bag in our trunk and slide back into my seat in the car. Driver/ Goon turns the key in his ignition and dims the headlights, and they leave first. We follow after two minutes. We do this most Tuesdays and know the routine by now. Why Tuesday? Because it fits his fucking schedule, and that's the answer we got.

Getting back to Chud's place feels like navigating the Mekong Delta, circa 1967, just with more acid, less rape, and the fact that we voluntarily do this — oh, and it's cold. Expecting Officer Charlie sporting a handlebar 'stache under a Saipan hat to pop out of every manhole, I envision my impending demise in an epic firestorm or, worse, being taken prisoner. But I won't let them get me alive. I'll go down swinging that straight razor for all I'm worth. I'll take a few of those mustachioed bastard-fucks with me.

Call it "being in the zone" — athletes pull off heroically inhuman acts of strength and skill. We drive a few blocks without looking suspicious.

My reverie is unceremoniously interrupted through a combination of the rapidly subsiding effects of cocaine and parking abruptly. We tread like fairy-tale mice at Christmas up the four flights of stairs, past the other apartments and into Chud's room.

> My head feels strange: empty. That can't be right.
> It has shit in it, I know that much for sure. I have
> thoughts like there should be three hundred and
> sixty degrees in a circle, and three hundred and
> sixty-six days on leap years. It's just that I've real-
> ized not a word has passed between us since the
> encounter, which lasted all of a minute, if that. I
> fleetingly wax metaphysical. I wonder if *I* actually
> exist; is there a *Me* aside from in my interactions
> with others? What language would I think in if I'd
> never learned one? Am *I* just a confluence of ex-
> ternal stimuli processed through a biological, von
> Neumann- or PDP-based, binary-logic assembly
> machine composed of neural switches? I don't
> think there's any sort of overarching meta-Self that
> *I* could actually identify with. I have as many differ-
> ent selves as I know people, one for each of them ...
> That's me, proud sponsor of whatever the fuck is
> going on here.

Wait, what the fuck *am* I talking about? Am I speaking to myself? Is this out loud? Can he hear me? No. I don't think so. Am I willing I into being — self-awareness? — in the absence of interactions with another algorithm analysis program?

Click.

The door shuts behind us and I toss the bag on the couch, collapsing beside it like a psychotropic body pillow. Chud turns on the vape while he packs a bowl. We're always careful to exhale through dryer sheets stuffed into an empty toilet-paper roll (lovingly termed "the sploof" and decked out as a dragon); it turns the telltale aroma of weed into a perfumed plume, indistinguishable from potpourri to your average ganja-ignoramus. Vaporizers don't smell as much as bongs or joints or pipes, but we still don't take any risks — in this respect, at least. He takes a few hauls, though it's not really cooking yet. Instead, we open up the bag and begin splitting the contents while we wait. It'll take a few hours to weigh everything, first to make sure we didn't get shorted on the order, then to divide it equally.

Inside, we find our leather-bound book full of LSD, lysergic acid diethylamide (code name: liquid soluble divinity), with an otherworldly, hypnotically designed cartoon character's face on each page; a ki of decent cocaine (purportedly Peruvian, but who knows in this economy); ten vacuum-sealed pounds of pot (five each of indica and sativa strains of varying qualities — there's something here for everyone); a brick of MDMA, straight from the chemistry team; five pounds of BC gold caps, purple-blue stemmed; an ounce of K; a gram of N,N-DMT, dimethyltryptamine (or "dreams made tangible"), for personal purposes; and fifty capsules of 2C-I for ... I dunno, fuck it, why not, right?

It's not the same every week. We do inventory checks on Saturday nights and place the order before we hit the bars. The runners can't always move everything we've got on hand. Sometimes there are special requests. It's simple supply and demand, really. This is an average-sized delivery and everything's for sale.

Lessons from Soulless
2010

"There are metrics of scale involved in this world of ours."

He doesn't smile. He doesn't look *at* us. He looks at us. What we are. Who we are. What we're worth. What he can take from us. What he can do to us. Chud and I do respect certain things. We shut the fuck up when Soulless is speaking.

"Selling more shit doesn't mean you're making more money."

That doesn't quite add up, but I know he likes dramatic pauses. I won't talk. His law's the law, even if we *act* lawless. He's the absolute inverse of Rodion Raskolnikov — he isn't desperate; he doesn't struggle with the morality of his actions; and *if* he were to kill, it would be intentional. He does not seek salvation. He's not the atonement type.

One night in grade twelve, my buddy wanted to go into High Park: some shit about his girlfriend dumped him and went to a party in the woods, and he just wanted the chance to talk to her again. I told him it might not be safe to stroll those paths past sundown, but he was adamant. Enter about twenty skinheads, our age, some of them mumble-mocking us with Eastern European accents, all of them wearing baggy white

T-shirts and closely buzzed haircuts ... or straight up shaved skulls. They start hassling my buddy (a short Trinidadian dude) and take his keys, wallet, and phone, threatening to leave him bleeding out in a leaf pile just off the path. They were a little less rough with me, patting me down instead of invading my pockets, demanding weed and money. I told my buddy to get the fuck outta there while I found the skinhead nearest to sobriety. I told him he was making a mistake. He asked me what I knew about mistakes. I dropped a few names I'd learned growing up in an Eastern European neighborhood — the sorts of names you'd expect to get a reaction from out of the next generation: nothing. He shoved me. I shoved back with one last name, [Soulless]. His dominant demeanour dissipated into deference. He shouted something to his cronies. There was a semblance of peace. My buddy came back from behind some trees to see what was going on, and one of the more inebriated skinheads punched him in the face, breaking his nose. My sober-ish skinhead counterpart quickly reprimanded the aggressor, kicking him and his clean white T-shirt into the dirt, all the while profusely apologizing to me. He yelled to the others to give my buddy back his keys, phone, and wallet (minus the money) and sent us on our way with pleas not to tell. Soulless was a name worth knowing.

Another time Soulless had offered me sex with a girl he'd been hanging out with. Forty bucks. That seemed low. I said no.

We're in Soulless's house in the suburbs of Toronto. His mom's in another room folding laundry; his toddler sister is playing in the hall. His bedroom door is ajar as he has a Tony Montana–style mound of coke on his desk. It's how he feeds the family. Admittedly, the pile isn't Hollywood sized, but that said, we've each had a few finger-sized lines out of it in celebration .

and are talking business at the conclusion of a merging of our distribution networks. We'll be in regular contact with him going forward. We're focused on the issues at hand.

We're also watching Soulless lift the rim of an inverted glass that's holding a captured spider he's dripped a drop of liquid LSD onto. He blows smoke into the cup, careful to fill it as much as possible. He closes the crystal cage and we watch the spider begin frantically, frenetically, frenziedly, and — I'm assuming — deeply psychotically zipping around the base of the glass, seeking the exit. Seeking, I'd say, any exit. But I ain't sayin' shit to Soulless. I'm always parsimonious with my words in his company. I don't even like spiders.

"So, you guys just bought a qp at eight-fifty. You sell it as half-quads for, what, forty?"

—Yeah. Or less if they're friends, y'know?

He looks *at* me again. He could take it all.

—I mean, like, there are a lot of factors, right? How well you know them. If they're good customers. If the market is flooded. All that shit.

"You charge what *you* want. Just pay me what *you* owe."

I gotta check myself. Sometimes I feel a rush of energy, and I just wanna smash this fuckwad through a window. It can happen in an instant. I'm a quick flip, not a dimmer. But … it's Soulless. He's like every Joe Pesci character rolled into one, except he doesn't make jokes, and he'd *actually* stab me to death with a pen if I ever made the connection for him.

—Yeah, man. Of course.

"If you followed my instructions, you'd be making more money selling a qp in hq's than a p in qp's. You'll make — or should make — more off that qp than I make off the pound it came from. Get it?"

—I guess. Yeah. So why do you sell more then?

"It's safer for me. I see four people. You see thirty-odd people. I'm covering my ass. I also don't have to hustle like you guys."

He looks at the spider. It's alive but not moving. Just there.

"I appreciate the hustle you guys have shown. That's why I made this deal. But see how that spider gave up?"

Chud answers, "Yeah?"

"He just couldn't hustle."

—We can hustle.

"Good. Comes a point you gotta realize that you can charge whatever you want with these cunts. I got a car from a crackhead for a five-rock once."

"Nice." Fucking Chud.

"What's this shit worth to people? What is the experience worth? You could buy it cheap as rancid pussy, sitting on a shelf for a year, then sell it in a second at twenty times its book value. Or you could pick product everyone likes and do it slow. Safe. Spread your holdings. That's my two."

—Well, we gotta build up to that level.

Chud chimes, "Yeah, man."

Soulless glances at the spider. He lifts the glass. It doesn't move. He nudges it. It just kind of shivers.

"Don't worry. I'll float you."

His palm slams down on the spider.

Retrospective Disclaimer

I've never claimed to be a good person. I like to think I am, but that's not enough to be a good person. I do things I regret instantly all the time. Maybe you can put it down to mental illness, but that in itself isn't enough to negate some of the things I do. I can be an outright outrageous douchebag. I'm not good with relationships or social interactions. Maybe my treatment of other people could be a little gentler, but I don't discriminate with my dislike. I hate everyone equally. I hate myself most. I don't think I'm a bad person, though. I guess you be the judge.

* * *

It's all there; I can finally exhale the stubborn bottom bit of breath I've been holding in for the last few hours. I hate the idea of having to call Soulless to tell him he's short. He always bitches about it and blames someone else. Bullshit, he's the CEO; he should accept responsibility for his lackeys the same way we do. At the end of the day, though, he scares the shit out of me. There's a pecking order here, and I've looked in his eyes and seen no reflections. Empty in there.

Chud lovingly places his share in one of his safes. We go back to my place and I do the same before we can head out for a night on the town. It's 11:00 p.m.

We get frisked at the door to the club, and the security guard finds the jackknife in my pocket but lets it pass. He knows who I am. Unless I'm much mistaken, he's got a nasty habit of his own and owes someone a few grand. He ushers us in, and I choose not to remind him. That's my runner's problem for giving credit to a fucking junkie.

Taking our seats right up in front of the stage, I place an order for tequilas with beer chasers. I recognize the girl performing; she works at the local Walmart and looks better with clothes on. By the scar on her abdomen, I'd say she has a kid — either that or she was a cutter, once upon a time. The fuck do I care? As long as she keeps shaking her bleached rosebud in my face, I'm happy.

When we pay for our drinks, I note the waitress's eyes. I forget about the state of my wallet — it looks like it has thyroid problems. She's got a bad poker face. A bad face in general, really, which could be why she's slinging sauce instead of slurping it.

She scuttles off to the professionals working the crowd, and next thing I know I'm talking to some Russian Twiggy look-alike about prices for a dance. She's as fresh off the boat as a barnacle, and I'm not sure if she's using her strong accent as a ploy to help her haggle, or if she legitimately just can't hold a conversation. Either way, she reminds me of my ex and she's wearing lingerie. I'm four shots and two beers in — so she has the upper hand.

She gives up trying to sell me on it, grabs my hand, and puts it on her tit, and I find myself following her to the backroom. I glance over to Chud, who winks at me like an epileptic staring at a coronal eclipse, a grin on his lips that would petrify Medusa. This man has evil thoughts — but I love him, for lack of a better word. It's not everyone that I can be myself with. As my father always told me in jest, "Good friends help you move, great friends help you move bodies." Not only would this guy help me move them, he'd make them. He'd grant dark wishes like a demented Kuklinski/genie hybrid. And he does it out of love — again, for lack of a better word. He'll be a lifelong friend. Nothing can break up our delinquent duo.

In the private lounge, the Russkeletor sits me down on a pleather couch. I hope they Lysol this shit. She drapes a bandana over my crotch, and then starts rubbing that general region with her entire body, writhing like she's in pain, which she very well could be, but as long as it's not from anything visible, I won't intrude.

The speakers are blasting some Top 40, ventriloquist dummy, make-believe rapper who rhymes poorly about drugs, guns, and hoes. Hey, at least he's making a living off the kids that actually believe him and buy this shit. Power to him.

The dance ends and the girl asks if I want another one. Tough call: variety is the spice of life. This is the best chance I've come across in a week for banking self-loathing I can use against myself if I ever sober up. I agree to one more dance and make a face like I'm doing her a favour. She wants to settle up on the last one before she starts. I get it. There are tricks to every trade, especially tricking. I nonchalantly flash the wad in my wallet as I whip out a twenty for her. It curls a little, almost into a tube, like muscle memory. The next song starts and she's made a quantum leap, suddenly pulling out all the stops.

She must want a third dance; I'm not sure yet if I do. I decide to test my luck. I start my fingertips behind her kneecap and work my way up. She doesn't object. A fat clit and a loose cunt. She's smooth. I suppose that's a job requirement. I lick my thumb and slip it in her asshole like I'm hitching a ride to horndog heaven and she takes this as a cue to whip off the bandana. I hear a zipping sound through the bass speakers.

She waits until I flop out and harden up enough to fill her hand with lacklustre libido — as firm as whatever flimsy ideology she follows on her days off — then she starts the bargaining again, all the while languorously working me like she's making bread from scratch. I'm not precisely a Herculean Pillar of wonder with women — especially after excessive narcotic abuse. Also I can tell she's enjoying this as much as stewing borscht. She briefly reminds me of a babushka, which doesn't help as I imagine her making cabbage rolls and recounting childhood traumas to disinterested Westernized grandchildren.

Where the fuck is my mind? Maybe this pixie can help me find the scattered shards of shrapnel of myself. Maybe she can explode my head in reverse.

No. Her technique needs improvement.

But she's playing Bambi-eyes. I do still want the money shot. Fuck, she's persistent … I'm not weak willed, but I'm still a heterosexual man with liquor in his system.

"One hundred! Plus dance."

—Only if you get the job done before the end of the next song. Deal?

"Sound like challenge."

I guess her accent *is* kind of cute — and I'm fascinated by her resemblance to someone I saw on a charity infomercial a few days ago. I hope I heard the price right. Meh, I'm not paying her till afterward anyway — she probably won't even be up to the task in hand, and who's she going to complain to? The bouncer that let me in? Ha! That guy can't even look me in the eye, let alone throw me out.

Fuck. She's really good at this. Where'd this come from? Who cares? Fuck it. Fuck-it. Fuckit. This is far, far better than I was expec-ec-ect-uhh, uh, uhhh …
My sahasrara swells and convulses in a nebulaic seizure of infinite ecstasy. Everything everywhere is white light that only I can *see and smell and touch and taste and hear and SHIT SHIT SHIT*: visible in a sense, but less than invisible to the senses.

She doesn't miss a beat or bat a Bambi eyelid, swallowing everything like it's Maxwell House. Holy fuck, this bitch just siphoned the last shred of sobriety out of me. She deserves more than a tip.

I get up, pay her through my post-orgasmic haze, and she leads me back to my seat before hitting up the next sucker. I manage to glimpse Chud heading to a different backroom with a tall, curvy girl wearing absurd stilettos and a Mrs. Mia Wallace wig. She stumbles a few times. He doesn't bother to help her up. He's cackling away instead and grabbing her ass. He must've had a few more shots during my absence. Usually, he's shy with women.

I've had people ask me how I live with myself. What kind of question is that? What else am I supposed to do with my "self"? Not live? I don't see the point in living if all you're looking at is the shadows on the wall. In fact, I tend to answer these people's questions with my own: What can *you* do? What changes can *you* effect when nothing you ever see *needs* changing? What do you *do*? Not that I'm out to save the world myself, or anything else as uppity — persnickety — as that. Shit, I just paid someone a hundred bucks to rent her digestive system. But at least I'm comfortable with myself. See, my partner and I, we're not *bad* people. We just do bad things particularly well. Whatever the fuck *bad* means in the first place. Who's to tell me what *bad* is? I built this shit out of my own will, like some sort of newfangled Nebuchadnezzar. A Zarathustra, forming a uniform morality in my own image. See me as evil if you will. I don't even see you. Nietzsche would be dying of maniacal laughter right now if he hadn't already.

I revert my attentions to the new girl onstage. Amateur night has its ups and downs. This is a down moment. I order more drinks. She's eyeing me, but she's still wearing pants, so I'm not about to get up there with her and make a donation. I just came, anyway. I like to choose my moments wisely, and my charities. The song ends and she steps down morosely. Nobody tipped her.

Really starting to feel the booze now. I excuse myself to go to the bathroom, where I bust out a line on the lid of the toilet, making sure to lock the door first. Even in a seedy environment like this, the management doesn't exactly approve of you doing blow in the open. I crush the rocks, chop it into a fine powder with playing cards (a jack and an ace — I don't really know why), roll up a hundred-dollar bill because I wanna feel like a big man, and I relish in the sting as it hits my sinuses: it's good. Good coke always smells like romaine lettuce and diesel to me. Then again, maybe I'm just fucked up. By the time I'm back at my seat I can't feel my front teeth and I'm clenching my jaw. This is really, really good — much better stuff than last time. Maybe even Peruvian ... does it matter?

Even though I just sat down, the next amateur is, again, far from inspiring, so I decide to go for a stroll.

I pass the bouncer on the way out and try to make eye contact. He used to buy off the owner of the club, like one of the girls; but then his intake surpassed his income. In order to keep his job — and likely other, more vital titles (like "mister") — he started digging a debt with my boy. I don't like his chances for once he hits bedrock bottom. This particular capo of mine has a dark side ... he likes the punishment and retribution aspect of this line of work more than anything, even the money. We all have our reasons. The bouncy castle of a bouncer studies his discount black leather shoes and pretends to pick something off his tie, which is immaculate already.

I open the door with a self-satisfied flourish and beeline for the circle of professional girls who are also indulging their relatively benign addictions. I pretend not to have a lighter in order to spark up conversation. They pass me a strike-anywhere but are uninterested in what I have to say, and unwilling to entertain my feigned interest in their formulaic, lackadaisical lives. So I go and lean against the wall, spitting occasionally and making a game of trying to start a puddle.

The door opens and the girls go in without a sideways glance. Yeah, fuck you, too. I wonder vaguely whether their conversation had been passing the Bechdel test before my arrival and consider that I may not have the healthiest sense of human decency.

"You good?"

Chud's lurching, fly down, toward me, lighting a joint with a lit cigarette already in his hand, and carrying a road beer. He's got a white moustache.

—Yeah. Good to drive?

"Won't kill anyone."

We hop in the car and pump some Ludwig van out of the subwoofer, as much to fuck with people's minds at three in the morning as because it's a beautiful sonata. I'm looking forward to getting home. I can see my Java-bear. She'll probably want a walk. This is the life. May it continue forever.

I'm lulled, despite the volume, to the lethargic, purgatorial cusp of sleep, then something shocks me out of my stupor — somehow, I have the momentary impression that my pants are full of bees. Gradually, reason reaches my unsettled psyche, and I realize it's just my phone: customers. It's a small chop, but a chop nonetheless. And we pass by this house on the way home anyhow. The strip club is on the outskirts of town. Probably some dumb-ass old rule about districting and morality. Chud lives close to the university, in a frat house he isn't a member of. I live about a five-minute drive down the road from him, in just ... well, a really unhealthy place and situation. These kids live right on the path. Always happy to make a quick buck.

—Dude, um ... umm ... Right! Hey, can we make a quick stop?

"Cool. Who?"

—Fucking wasps, man. Fuckin' wasps ...

"Huh? You fryin' or somethin'?"

—Like chicken, bro ... Special, secret blend. Herbs. Spices. Shh ...

* * *

The room oozes bad karma and worse habits — I'm drawn to it like a fawn to the salt stains of the highway before being smote by hallucinogen-addled teenagers on an intergalactic voyage at warp speed inside of a fetus-coloured Pontiac Sunfire.

I push the door open to be met by shit-faced grins, gawking at me through the topsy-turvy, swirling, curling, opalescent eddies of cyanic, sterling silver–pearl smoke. Tangy traces of tequila tickle my nostrils, mixed with the citrus elements of a sativa-dominant strain of cannabis. This is the smell dreams are made of.

Assuming a position on the couch between a dreadlocked trust-fund artist and a pro bono nude model watching pornography blooper videos, I rummage in my pocket for a second before extricating a Baggie full of little Baggies full of these people's main nutrient source: drugs. Fuckloads of drugs.

To tell the truth, these people sicken me. These little encounters give me the heebie-jeebies. They represent everything I stand against; they are everything I oppose — like a mirror image inverted. These sheep in wolves' clothing, though, are my bread and butter. Pseudo-intellectual sorts that discuss the comparative merits of Kierkegaard and de Beauvoir while puffing on hash-laced hookahs and sipping Chimay spiked with MDA, in between bouts of snorting cocaine cut with a proprietary blend of aniracetam, novocaine, noopept, and other fillers. I bet they've never even heard of Levinas.

—That'll be two-fifty.

Dreadlocks passes me two hundred-dollar bills and a fifty. The thought of this kid in patched jeans and a threadbare sweater owning a bank account seems odd, until I remember what he told me last time I was here:

"Yeah, my dad's one of the top criminal defence lawyers in Toronto."

—Cool.

I relish the idea of Dreadlocks, Pro Bono, and the rest of them shoving expensive baby laxatives up their noses. I complete the transaction and ready myself to leave.

—Enjoy your shit.

* * *

Finally home, I try to pass out for about half an hour but the coke's still got me buzzing, so I go back downstairs and turn on the TV. Java's looking at me. I look back. I'm not in any state to take her down the street to the park for a walk, so I let her out in our backyard. It's a two-storey house with three bedrooms and a backyard for two people and the pets. Under nine hundred a month. Gotta love small-town schooling. Java poops and comes back in. I'm not cleaning it up. I head back to the telly. There's nothing good on — not surprising at this hour. I go to one of my safes, open it up, and grab a fresh sheet of acid. This was a one-off sheet, meaning I got it alone, not as part of a larger volume or "book;" the trademark art is all in black and white and makes a bizarre maze with no way to the centre. Intriguing. I carefully cut out five tabs and pop them under my tongue, letting adolescent nostalgia overwhelm me as I reminisce with myself, led by a subtle, bitter, metallic taste of this liquid soluble divinity. I go back to the TV and pop in a DVD: *Apocalypse Now*.

TWO

Early 2017

Where has the time gone? I mean, you hear it all the time growing up, but it doesn't really register. Then you take a bunch of drugs for the first time in your early teens, when your mind is still elastic, and you realize time is elastic, too: the same amount of time can stretch way, way out until it no longer even seems like the same material, or it can spring back to normal in the instant you sober up. Or you can black out and lose huge tracts of your life to someone else in the driver's seat — someone you hadn't realized was even in your vehicle.

Once you stop taking the drugs, time doesn't seem to stretch the same way. Maybe that's why I never really stopped. I mean, I slowed down, for sure, but I never full-stopped — never put a period on that sentence. Old age and incapacitation and mortality ... even dementia ... seem so much further away when you're wasted.

I'm in a curious place now. I'm genuinely trying to steer clear of most of the old street drugs. I even quit smoking — on the e-cig option at present, except when I have to go to the hospital now and then and can only get nicotine patches and that numbing gum. The five years between that fateful dawn of fights and furies and now — it's been full of far-out and fucked-up experiences. I did fentanyl before the headlines. Buying pounds of mushies without the customer base any-more — just, literally, eating my debt. I've popped a planet's worth of Xanax. I've been prescribed almost every antidepres-sant and second-generation antipsychotic on the market, and a few that lean into that scary first-generation collection. My suicide attempts have been numerous and largely unmemor-able, though not largely untraumatic.

The last was in late September of 2016, in the triage ward of the decaying and dying College Street location of CAMH (Centre for Addiction and Mental Health) in Toronto, which I suspect is haunted by the ghosts of former patients suffering all sorts of mind-ravaging intergenerational, post-mortem traumas. If the nurse who untied the bedsheet from my throat is reading this, I'd like to extend a true thanks. I owe you this book. I'm in a new program now, the Transitional Care Program, which I simultaneously hope and doubt will be my last. My family, friends, and partner are all (naturally, I'd say) worried about me — but I feel good today, for the first time in what feels like the first time.

I have a girlfriend. Not the one you met earlier. This one's a keeper. I mean, sure, we still fight ... more than either of us would like, but that's what you've got to expect in a relationship where both participants have difficulties distinguishing reality from perception. The love is there, though. She's stuck with me through so much that I can't envision a life without her; though, in those darker moments, I often fear it.

I wish I knew what's wrong with me — what, exactly, is my major malfunction? I'm sure the drugs haven't helped, but there's something else there, something that's always been there. Since it first came into existence, my psychiatric file has had an uncompromising question mark next to the diagnosis, and I feel like if I just knew what that question mark represented, I'd be in a better position to address it.

A large part of the theory behind magic — real magic, not just sleight of hand — is the knowledge of the *true names* of things. When you can name something, you have a power over it. I wish I knew my name.

THREE

Retrospective on 2008:
Acid Flashback

Skittles didn't know his name.

Skittles wasn't my friend, despite his desire to be. I made that clear. We were dormmates, and he hung around ... but he rubbed too many people the wrong way, and he creeped out the girls down the hall. Still, living two doors down from someone in crammed university lodgings only affords you so many ways to avoid others, and at the end of the day, I'm an ambivert and can be somewhat of a people person, so socializing does wonders for my mood. Everyone else was busy doing something to do with being at school — studying, dating, taking exams, playing ultimate frisbee — all the sorts of shit they put in the pamphlets, but I felt like going off menu. Skittles's door was open.

I popped my head around the corner to look in. His half of the room looked like the scene out of *A Beautiful Mind* where they discover John Forbes Nash Jr. has gone totally batshit. Bits of string, newspaper clippings, tape stuck to tape stuck back onto a roll of tape. Weird dude. He was sitting on his bed. Little guy — maybe five foot six or so, like, 130 pounds ... wild, untamed, hobbit-lookin' curly hair. His clothes were basic. Baggy. Hoodie and jeans, no labels, no logos. We shared a belief in not advertising other people's brands for free.

—Hey, man. Sayin'? What you got going on for the next twelve hours?

This was a stupid move even on the surface of it. Don't take mind-warping substances with people you don't know very well, or people with deep-seated issues you don't intend to help them with, or people who outright bug you. But I was "desperate."

Skittles's access to drugs was pretty much dependent on mine, with me being the resident plug, grabbing products from Toronto that were hard for the local populace to procure. He was enamoured by the concept of psychedelia. He'd pepper me with questions about what to expect from a new experience, or what mixed well with what, or what the best music was for each drug. He'd ask strange questions about what it would be like to kill someone or die on acid. Weird kid. My castaway comments were his forming events, and the course of his lifespan was my present tense.

"Ha ha ha. My man. You know I'm down. Is it the same batch?"

When he laughs, it sounds sarcastic, but it's not. It's just him.

—Um, I've got two tabs left from the old sheet, then a fresh page that's supposedly even stronger but still has the same artwork.

"Cool. Cool. Let's make it a special one. How are we gonna do it?"

As a veteran psychonaut, I felt comfortable jumping right on in with whatever was thrown at me. I felt particularly confident that I could ride out the high tides held on these cute little smiley-face tabs, with each smiley face making up the larger smiley face that dominated the front of the next page on deck. But Skittles was still new to the game, so I suggested he take it slow.

Skittles

```
I handed you a half smile, then
the fellow followed, like a friend

would make you whole, & might help
change our strange directions. We'd
  dealt

with 'cid enough to know those signs
of when a good time hit its decline

& rough trips were in need of abrupt
  ends:
how well-worn laugh lines cut, too
  deepened

just before leaving, or seizing
in place, faking faces not even

reflections could lessen the horror of —
though, your lips sat so still at the
  corner
```

```
as they ordered, "One more smile."
My story-less book stored another tile

we tore out of the untouched page
which, being fresh, had no gauge

&, God bless, held your name on it:
you bit into bitterness, a little
    demonic

pop-culture happiness icon, an edible
hieroglyph with a nearly identical

expression second-guessing itself
as you'd stuck to your gums, unfelt

until at last that lilt crept up some
    undone tongue
it hung from reason's wilting prison
    windowpane
```

Then, suddenly, all serious:

"I'm seeing things, guys. Please, help me stop this. Please. It keeps speaking to me about going insane, and it's saying I can't get back to the same place ever again, and I've snapped my last strap, and I'm fucking scared. Go away, man. I'm done here, since this isn't real. It isn't real and nothing is as real as feeling this. Guys, I'm not prepared for the *true* psychedelic experience."

The next day Skittles hadn't come down. He tried to smoke some pot to cool his head, but that was a bad call all around. Cannabis potentiates a lot of psychedelics. Soon Skittles was complaining about hands coming out from beneath his bed to pin him down and purple pterodactyls outside his window.

Two days later and he was gone. He'd called his parents out of desperation and told them what he'd done and what was happening. They'd whisked him away to the hospital.

I was so relieved.

When Skittles came back, he was definitely different. Quiet. Withdrawn and reclusive and not quite "there." Permanently dilated pupils drifted amid his freckle mask. He had a light year–long stare about him. One night he showed up to a party and smoked weed again for the first time since his episode. He began speaking in riddles, then gibberish word salad, then not even English. It sounded like what I imagine Parseltongue must sound like. We had to carry him out of the party and into a cab as he writhed and screamed at the universe. After that I didn't see him again. He dropped out of school for good.

Years later I met with my first roommate from university for nachos and a pint, and he filled me in on the rest of the story. Eventually, Skittles jumped off a bridge. He was schizophrenic. The acid sped up or exacerbated the process. I felt, and still feel, like a non-fictional Duddy Kravitz encouraging the epileptic Virgil to drive, except Virgil lived while Skittles didn't. I guess I have to honour his wishes. He *didn't* want to live, it seems. Is "schizophrenia" a *true name*? Skittles, I'm so sorry.

FOUR

Retrospective on 2012: Fallout

Yeah, that definitely wasn't LSD. It wasn't even in that whole generally safe lysergic class. My best guess is that it was the vivid fever-dream/nightmares of an unmedicated schizophrenic condensed onto perforated rice papers. I will likely never be the same, and I'm not sure whether that makes me happy, sad, or one of those new emotions I feel now that defy linguistic interpretation. It's part of the reason I have no tattoos. Got plenty of scars and fucked-up colours in my skull already; don't need 'em on my skin.

To be entirely honest, I can't exactly recall what happened that morning. There are several accounts: the legal documents, the psychiatric reports, my ex's three or four conflicting stories from various points in her grieving process, and my unsound memories. I'll here recount the version that doesn't make me feel like following Skittles off the edge of a bridge. It's probably not entirely true or accurate or coherent, but that's something I'll have to atone for at some point in the future, every day of my life.

We were fighting — had been for a few months. But we were still living together, for reasons that, in retrospect, seem unfathomable. I was supposed to be moving out later that day — my folks were on their way to get me and the last of my stuff.

As has been alluded to, I was tripping unprecedented balls in the living room. To calm myself, I took a gram of MDMA, which didn't work as well as I'd thought it should. I just wanted something positive to hold on to. I had the knife in my pocket, and I was as unstable as a feral stallion, to say the least. I thoughtlessly pulled the knife out of my pocket and started to doodle in the crook of my left forearm with the blade, tracing veins and building pressure to take the plunge. The knife was rusty and dull, covered in sticky drug residue and dried blood, and wasn't keeping the lines of my drawing as crisp and clear as I'd wanted. I decided to sharpen it. My ex was screaming and crying and saying unintelligible things. I wanted some peace and quiet, that's all.

—Either shut the fuck up and leave me alone, or I swear to God I'll jam this fucking knife square in your face. One of us has to go. Make the call.

That seemed to work. She got her phone and left the room, and all was well for a while. I heard the door slam and footsteps through the window running to the park down the street. I went to the kitchen to get my blade sharpener and had a smoke on the porch while I scraped the edges clean before making another attempt at my little piece of inner arm artwork. Java was barking, for some reason.

Apparently, though, she'd been yelling for help up and down the street, called 911, and gotten her say in before me.

I first noticed the police when they threatened to shoot me. That snapped me out of it. Didn't even see the cars or hear the screeching tires or comprehend the neighbours peering through their drapes, but I clocked the six pistols trained on me and heard their urges to discard my weapon. I let the cigarette drop from my lips into the bushes in front of me, not trusting my hands to do their job correctly. Totally forgot about the knife, back in my pocket.

To their credit, they seemed pretty decent about the whole thing. Asked me if the handcuffs were too tight and if they could enter the house, not that they needed my permission (luckily nothing was found … there was enough stuff around the house to keep me in government lodgings for multiple lifetimes).

"Hey, kid, can you understand me?"

I had no fucking idea what was happening aside from noticing the phenomenological fractals cracking and fraying the fracking sky open. They were distinctly separate from me, and not anything I could construe as "regular reality," but drew all my attention inexorably upward and twisting around. I felt phenomenally illogical as the spinning, psychotically summoned tripartite designs of triskelions twirled and unfurled into infinities of each other, reminding me of my Celtic heritage. Odd time for that. I wasn't in the right mindset to be arrested at that precise moment.

—Yeah.

They read me my rights. I think.

An unclaimed question appeared in my ear. "What's the charge?"

I didn't hear the answer. I wouldn't have understood anyway. They took me to the hospital in handcuffs. I was *that* guy in the triage. Blood tests. Shit, I was fucked.

"There's nothing acutely wrong with him, aside from the toxicology, but we're sending him to Homewood for observation until he can stand trial."

That didn't sound good.

And then it was off to the Homewood Health Centre — the mental asylum. My memory from this whole period is fuzzy. Actually, I can barely remember any of it. I think this is where I got my call.

—Hey, Dad. How's it going?

"We're OK. What's going on with you?" They must have noticed something was up when they got a collect call from a mental asylum.

—I'm not so good. I got arrested.

Silence.

—Dad?

"Yes. I'm here. I love you. What happened?"

I told him … or tried, at least. I did my best to get my point across without admitting my guilt or, y'know, mentioning that I'd been more than reasonably deep in the drug game. I thought I could still salvage all this. I was also still somewhere past the atmosphere. The drugs still had me … I wasn't clear.

"And what are the charges?"

Good question. I ask the orderly monitoring my phone call. "Attempted murder."

Oooh fuck.

"We'll get a lawyer and be there tomorrow. Try not to say anything."

Bed Bound

I'm tied to a bed of sorts. Like a doctor's bed, not the type that invites rest. There's paper involved. It's white and sterile here. Tools, no toys. A lady in a white coat with a clipboard is talking to me. She's not alone. She's in the room. No, she's not, actually. That was a trick. She's on an intercom. She's behind a glass screen reinforced with mesh wire. Why? There's a painting in the hallway behind her. It's not a bad painting. A lady bending down to give a child something. It looks like Paris in the twenties. I'm strapped down. I lock eyes with her. She looks at her clipboard and her ponytail bobs playfully, then stops. She's focused on the clipboard, not me.

"Can you tell me how you're feeling?"

Man, I'm tripping balls. Did I take it all? I can't recall. I can't remember anything at all.

—Good.

"Can you tell me where you are?"

I hear a voice. It's in the painting? Or the hall? Not in my ears. No. Still in my noggin', though. Not through the wall. It's not a choice. Is this the voice of God? I respect it now. Capital *G*. Should I rejoice? It's not the right time to have God foisted on me by the drugs. I'm far too flawed to be awed at the moment. I should hide inside the cloister of the moisture fogging up my opened eyes. I should pretend to be blind. Or deaf instead, I guess. Yes. Or no, actually. It's God, after all. It can call me on my bullshit.

—I'm in detention.

"You're at the Homewood facility. You aren't well. You *are* safe. Can you tell me why you're here?"

I'm too odd to be appreciated by God. I'm not chosen. My body's contorted uncomfortably with the dysesthesia I've impudently created. My God speaks. I nod in akathisia. I understand. I understand it all. I weep. I try to stand up to applaud. But what? What was it God said? *"Don't worry. Everything's gonna be all right. Don't worry. You'll survive the night."* Sounds like a knock-off Bob Marley. That's all it commits to. One night? I have my fucking life to worry about and it gives me one fucking night? I realize God's not worth crying over. What a slipshod fraud of a god. God doesn't deserve applause.

"Sir, do you know why you're here?"

I've trod beyond these thoughts before, though. Beyond beyond. Beyond beyondness and beyond. Fuck Buzz Lightyear; I'm on Alderon. I've blown apart and gone far gone. Gone on and on and on. And more. This is stranger than a chamber full of chambers full of Edgar Allen Poes, and darker than the raven sitting on his chamber door.

—I took too much drugs …

"That's likely. But do you remember what happened next?"

What's with the floor? It's shifting shape. One second curvy, the next it's flat. I can't tell what the fuck it's moving for. And, what's the "what" in "what the fuck"? Like, what the fuck's the "what"? What's up with that? And what the fuck is going on with mysticism? Why does it rhyme with pessimism and ellipsism? Am I just tripping or is this some wisdom? Am I a living puppet or is this ventriloquism? Where's Geppetto in this mix? And can she see my nose as it grows?

—The police came. They threatened to kill me.

"They wouldn't have threatened to kill you. They may have asked you to do something or they'd be forced to fire on you, but they wouldn't threaten to kill you."

I test the straps around my wrist. They force my rest.

I'm "word of god" verbal-vibe soliloquy-style fighting, solo in the dojo of my mind. I'm Neo, the hero and zero in one. But I gotta pick something. It's one or the other and I can only pick the numbers. I can't run from this. I Humperdinck myself the way I fucking think — musically drunk, but how was that done? I hardly drink, except when I drink rum. I fucking stink. I'm fucking dumb. I'm feeling so low I need reminding to live a little, "yolo."

—Are you going to kill me?

"No. You aren't going to die here. We're here to help you."

I need to know exactly what kind of guy I am. The type to take the whole world on with a Cerebro-form of bolo knife. I'm so psychokinetically capable right now Magneto couldn't make me let it go to save his life. I'd save his soul pro bono then sell it back to Hell, like, "Hell no, my dear fellow!" I'd even blow the bellows on the fire. Fuck bonobo living — I'm not as peaceful. I need to make a living. I'll parse this evil planet into parts to eat it piecemeal. Everything has earned my ire. I'm aching for upheaval.

—I'm innocent. I just took drugs.

I'm still. I'm still stuck in my pill-filled skull. I'm fucked in this void. I look nullified to any onlookers. A rebooting droid. A clogged pressure cooker I toyed with naively. I'm lost in a hologram, needing a hospital. I'm in a hospital. I'm in a hospital? This doesn't feel safe. This doesn't feel real.

"Do you remember why the police were called?"

I detect false confidence. Like, "I'm bolo," as in, "be on the lookout" for the five-o popo, just kids who graduated from popping their polos to pieces off for the fun of it, those mofos tearing up the momentary "all of creation" I've made for myself in my own imagination. The imagination the whole world should take in. I hate them. They shill shit and kill trips. But that's their business.

—Because they're afraid of drugs.

"I think there must be more to the story than that. Can you tell me what happened?"

—Yeah.

What the fuck's my brain saying? Is this praying? More like a malaise of unamazing. This is nonsense. This is so non-Zen. Just ignore me. This is beyond sense. Where is my conscience? I have one. Honest.

"Can you tell me more? I want to help."

Suspend belief in my disbelief of myself and be felt. I know I can do it. I know that I need it. I need help.

But honesty has too often gotten the best of me.

—No.

She passes the clipboard to someone else as she turns away from me, her ponytail waving goodbye.

"I don't think we can do much for him. I'm afraid to medicate him. I guess — maybe time?"

They walk away. I can't hear, though. The intercom is off. They turned it off just before they left. Why'd they leave it on so long?

* * *

Before my parents arrived, I was transferred to an isolated holding cell in the city's police headquarters. No visitors. I was awaiting what I understood to be a pretrial sort of thing ... I'd been assigned a public defender. Where were my parents?

I would be held in the police headquarters over the weekend until my pretrial on Monday. But I couldn't stay there over the weekend. The weekend held something special in store for me.

FIVE

2012: Lock-Up

"Bend over. Spread your cheeks. Cough. Go to the next station."

"Put your thumb on this ink. Roll it around. Press it to this paper. Go to the next station."

"Look right here. Don't smile. Turn left. OK, turn right. OK, go to the next station."

I feel like telling me not to smile was either a vestigial sense of normalcy from the guard's life outside the walls, where people smile, or a nonchalantly tossed out dig at another junked-up criminal nuisance case.

Weekend holding at Maplehurst Penitentiary. The Milton Hilton. They shipped me out in a court services armoured truck with a few other fuckups, and I was sent to sweat out my demons and numerous, varied addictions in the suicide ward on a concrete bed with no blanket.

The metal is what I remember most. Metal everywhere. Cold. Hard. Sharp-edged. Even the floor felt like metal as I rested my forehead against it in some newly found belief, a born-again perverse form of prayer. The other guys in the truck were metal. Not, like, Whitesnake, Metallica, or Guns N' Roses shit … they were made of iron. And I was soft. I know that now. I knew that then. I was just afraid to admit it to myself, let alone them.

I wouldn't mind getting hold of my mugshot. It would've made a conversation-starting author photo for the back of this book. Instead I'm stuck with the only headshot I have, from a food, jobs, and clothing drive at a mental hospital.

Next station.

"Why are you here?"

—Umm … I dunno. I got arrested.

He looked vexed, but I think I got him to crack a smile. Hey, I still had it, even under duress. Sure, that'll come in handy.

"What did you get arrested for?"

—I'm not quite sure. Umm, there were a bunch of things they mentioned, but it was all a bit hectic. There was a great deal of consternation, and I'm not quite myself at the moment. Sorry. I think it's attempted murder?

That time he laughed. His desk-jockey job jowls jiggled to his giggle.

"You must be the most polite kid here. You're gonna get torn apart."

He went to some other guards, and they shuffled some papers and talked, but I couldn't hear them over the sounds of my fellow degenerates being processed. One of them laughed, too. The guard came back after about five minutes.

"OK, just follow the lines and the guard will put you in a holding cell."

No laughter anymore as I shambled into a room about one hundred square feet with about twenty other guys in it. I sat down between a clean-cut fellow with a crisp white button-up shirt and polished black-leather shoes. I'm guessing drunk driving. On my other side was Big Red. That's legitimately what he told me to call him. Just shy of seven feet, bald with a big ginger beard, and probably a few stone over three hundred pounds. He looked like if Buddha got into survivalism and joined a militia. Though, at the time he was tranquil, like the cell was his summer home.

Now I just have to say here, for the sake of transparency, that I have very little memory of any of this. You're reading a reimagining based on a true story. I was coming down from an Ozzy Osbourne's worth of brain damage and coming off a Keith Richards amount of extremely dependence-inducing drugs. I should've, by all rights, disappeared from the face of the earth, like a Keith Moon.

This was a new low point in life. I was physically weak. I was scared. I was solo. I knew I was in there with a bunch of guys who'd shred me if they found out why I was really there (a lot of these dudes had daughters in the real world). Sure, I played hard while I was free to. And I'd done some shit, yeah. Other people were scared of me. But I was fucking terrified in there. And I was *still* tripping far too much to be caged. Coming off drugs can be as trippy as getting on them.

There were things I'd been prepared for about the experience from stories, scared-straight visitors to my elementary schools, and the TV series *Oz*, which I'd ironically finished watching not even a month before. But nothing can quite prepare you. For instance, I knew from casual conversations with drug dealers that you don't call someone a *goofball*. I didn't exactly know why, I just knew not to do it. However, I didn't know to stay away from any iteration of words starting with *g-o-o-f*. I fucked up. When the other guys asked what I'd done, I said that I'd goofed my life and gotten arrested. I thought I was being conservative with the whole avoiding "I threatened my ex with a knife to the face" play. But my statement earned me a lot of cold looks and a moment of silence until the meaning of the word (a *goofball* is a pedophile), and thus the situation, cleared itself up. It could've gone differently, and it wouldn't take much in this little room for anything to go wrong.

Where even was I? I'm pretty sure it was prison, but I was still wearing my street clothes. I think. Actually, I can't remember that, either. I'm sorry. It felt like jail. It looked and seemed like the jail I'd come to expect from TV, but I'd come there from ... where had I come there from again? Doesn't prison have jumpsuits and, like, proper loneliness — as in, being solitary *and* alone?

Time passed in a plodding sort of way. I don't think I was actually in there for that long, but it felt like enough. We all just tried passing the hours. I learned of various ways to open a beer bottle with a gun, or a Coke bottle if you're showing the kids. I guess you gotta stay positive, right?

* * *

Fuck. Keep it cool, man. Just breathe.
It fucking stinks in here.

The precariously easy vibes are abrasively ended when a new inmate is ushered into our cell. He rushes over to a normal-seeming dude tucked away in the corner looking scared as shit and starts smacking the bejesus outta him, screaming bloody murder.

"You fucked me man! You fucked me. You're a rat! See this guy? This guy right here? He's a fucking rat! And he's a dead man. You hear me? You're a fucking dead man! I'm gonna fucking kill you, fucking rat shit fuck!"

Whack. Whack. Whack.

Where are the guards?

Whack. Whack. Whack.

The new guy's wearing a fucking track suit. Chav as shite. Platinum blond hair, buzzed on the sides, short on top ... skinny dude. Bulging junkie veins in a child's arms. Purple spots on the insides of his elbows. Black tats from his wrists to his ears. The guy getting beaten looks like an elementary school teacher ... mushroom haircut. Nothing out of place, apart from the glasses getting smacked off his face.

Whack. Whack. Whack.

"You're a fucking dead man, you pussy! Ima gut you, bitch! You're dead!"

Whack. Whack. Whack.

He could've been a dead man by now. A guard shouts around a corner.

"Hey, you in there! Calm down! Shut the fuck up!"

Chav walks to the other side of the room, across from Mushroom Haircut, and stares at him. I mentally prepare for a prison group Holmgang ... like, a hazing ritual or something. A "beat-in" with shivs. Brazen poundings must be a fairly regular — or at least acceptable or somewhat anticipated — occurrence, since Big Red sort of breaks the tension and asks the room in general if anyone likes heroin. I can't imagine there are many government institutions where you can toss that question out and still be welcome in the building. I guess this *is* the place. I'm still shit-scared of everyone (except Mushroom Haircut and Drunk Driver), not least of all the seemingly placid Big Red, but through the chemically induced crumbling caverns of my cranium comes a desperate answer. Desperate to connect with a safe audience. Desperate to connect me to the safety of that audience. I need a guardian right now.

—I mean. Yeah, I like heroin.

His Norse god–sized head turns with its barren peak and bountiful beard, and a full berserker-style gaze meets mine as he cracks a smile.

"Settle a debate. Heroin or oxys?"

—Oxy.

"Naw, man. Oxy's got no personality. Just high. Heroin, it's all different err'y time. Batches, y'know? Like weed."

—Yeah, man, true. But you have no idea how strong that heroin is. I like not dying when I'm just trying to chill. I really prefer Dilaudids.

If I show some sort of higher knowledge of opiates, maybe I can ingratiate myself with this guy. At least, that's where my mind was going with this.

He giggles like an Ent. Long, slow, ponderous, and with purpose. There's a bark to it.

"Right. Oh, fuckin' right, I forgot Dilaudids. We should meet on the outside."

Doubtful.

—I'm not sure when I get out.

"Nobody is."

* * *

Dinner was food. It came with a peach cup and I don't like peaches, so I offered it to Big Red, who told me in hushed tones never to give up a piece of your hot meal, even voluntarily, since any signs of weakness stir up the predatory instincts. Blood on the wind. Better to waste it than give it, or have it taken.

Soon I was separated from the safety of Big Red and sent to the suicide-watch ward.

I was led into a corridor of solitary units, all on one side, if I remember anything correctly. I didn't bother to look right and see how far they stretched, one door every ten feet or so, going on for … a while. I'd been ushered into the first cell in front of me and walked into it through an opened-up slab of steel on hinges. It shut like a sarcophagus.

I punched the door, and it had the same effect as a dead man punching his coffin lid, except I could still feel the instant pain in my fist. Bruised knuckles. Red palm. No blood. No cracked bone. Guess I couldn't be that upset. Maybe I didn't have it in me. To my right was a wall, beyond which I knew nothing. To my left was a wall with another dude behind it, I assumed.

I got a gown that sort of felt like the lead gowns you wear while getting an X-ray. It was as indestructible as everything else in the cell: a raised concrete bed with no pillows or mattress or sheets, in case I MacGyver'd a noose out of the fabric. There were no bars, no natural light, just that solid steel door with several layers of locks and a slot — two-ish inches high, six-ish wide — to look out at the empty hall and scream through.

I called out for the guards, but nobody came.

I don't even know what I'd have asked for. *Can I have a blanket? Can I talk to a doctor? Can I go home?*

* * *

My neighbour is talkative, after a while. I guess he heard me scream myself quiet before he piped up: "So, what'd you do?"

Shit, it really echoes in here. There is absolutely nothing soft to soak up the sound. Metal, concrete, and men. His voice is smoke. He was talking through his two-ish inch–high slot and it was bouncing off the wall across from us and through my two-ish inch–high slot with ease. If there are guards out there, they can hear all this. As well as my screams.

—Attempted murder.

"Oh shit, bruh. Tell me about it."

I don't want to tell him about it. But I sort of need to say something. I don't know how long I'll be here.

—Man, I was on mad drugs and shit. I don't really know what happened. I'm still tripping.

"Is that why you're on suicide watch?"

—Maybe.

"So ... would you actually do it? Suicide? Or are you just here to get away from the other guys? Scared?"

Both? I don't know.

—Yeah, man.

"Sheeeit. You sound young, bruh. Where you from?"

I don't want to give this random dude on suicide watch in prison my fucking address. I don't even want to be talking. I want to scream and punch soft things.

—Twenty-two, bro. Old enough for this shit, apparently. High Park.

"Oh, my cousins grew up near to you."

I don't need the family connection. I don't want to take any of this back with me. We chat about the cherry blossoms, nonetheless, and playing shinny on Grenadier Pond. I'm crying, but he can't see it. I make sure he doesn't even hear it.

"You got a girl, son?"

—Not anymore, man.

He smiles to himself, but of course I hear it:

"My wife's gonna be sooo pissed."

* * *

That's about all I remember from the suicide-watch block.

After the weekend I was sent back to the jail in the police headquarters. It was time to go to the courthouse to figure out what in the fuck the rest of my life would look like. I piled into another fortified truck with some other guys, and we speculated on what we'd do when we got out.

"I'm gonna get clean."

"I've got a big job set up"

—I have no clue.

"I'm gonna find that fucker, Greg, and throw him off a fucking 401 overpass. He squealed on me over an onion. Would any of you flip for an onion? Who the fuck can't handle that?"

An onion is an ounce of cocaine. You'd still do hard time. For some people that's a tough call. The conversation ended.

Court made me feel anxious. I was hoping for whatever miracle would get me a bed, bail, and a frail sense of freedom, even if it was one I could hang myself with.

I saw my parents for the first time in what seemed like a paradigm. They were reserved. This felt more like an interview than a family reunion. Yeah, right, keep trying to hide that shame. It's coming out eventually, I know it.

We got a lawyer. A sleazebag. And that's me saying it. He talked to judges; he talked to prosecutors; he had lunch; he played golf. My dad paid a retainer fee, and the charges dropped from attempted murder, to assault with a deadly weapon, to uttering a death threat … yeah, death threat sounds right. That *is* all I did. I have no fucking clue where this "attempted murder" bullshit came into it.

I reached out to any upstanding professionals I knew for reference letters: doctors, lawyers, teachers, etc. My ethics professor said something along the lines of "Good luck with your job applications" in their accompanying email.

The judge read out a long list of all the drugs I had in my system when I was arrested, with my parents sitting in the courtroom, and I wouldn't have thought it was something you could walk away from. I can't remember exactly what was in the toxicology report, but I know there was cocaine, amphetamines, several forms of opioids, MDMA, benzodiazepines, ketamine, alcohol, cannabis, and a few others. I wasn't in great spirits.

My parents met me outside the courthouse and took me home after. They weren't happy.

I was banned from the city I'd gone to university in, except for legal meetings and court appearances, which included seeing *her* again, with her family.

There was a moment in court, about a year after the initial event. It was weird. I'd been to an earlier court appointment where it all seemed fairly cut and dry. I was being charged with uttering a death threat. I was prepared for that. Then in my final court appearance (where I was feeling fairly confident), the prosecution approached the judge, talked for a minute or two, and then the judge called my ex to talk in private. What the fuck was this?

"The prosecution has made me aware of certain aspects of this case I had not been informed of. This young lady has made some very serious claims."

I exchanged looks with my mom. Ever the protector of the family, she'd even once followed me outside in winter, shoeless along the snow and ice, to coax me home when I'd tried to run away one day. She is familial love incarnate — if a tad unforgiving and blunt, at times. I come by it honestly. Bless her.

She whispered with apprehension: "What could she be saying?"

I didn't feel like telling my mom any of the various incriminating things she could be saying.

The judge continued. "Unfortunately, the new information cannot be used in this trial; though, if it were, I am certain the defendant would not fare as well."

What the fuck did she say? That I was a drug dealer? Probably. But was that it? Was that enough to make this judge turn cold as Arctic coprolite? Or did she say something more insidious? I didn't do anything. I swear. I didn't do anything. Except threaten to kill her, I guess.

I got probation, community service, and a conditional discharge. A slap on the wrist. No criminal record, thank the lords. Then home. Home to my family, my shame, my temporary sobriety. Home to consolidate my various peaces. Home to what and where I needed to be.

My dad clapped me on the shoulder as I was getting into the car.

"It'll all work itself out someday. Maybe this will make an interesting chapter in a book."

The jovial sentiment wasn't homogenous, though. My parents were very serious about certain things. That quarter million I had stashed away in a safe for a rainy day? I still don't know where it is. I suspect at the bottom of Lake Ontario, getting the fish fucked up off the numerous substances I had tucked away in there along with the bills. They had the safe. They took it to "keep it safe." They had the key. But knowing them, they wouldn't want to be party to anything illegal. Fuck, my dad won't even ride his bike on the sidewalk. No, wherever it is, it's gone.

Chud visited me a few months after I got home. My parents didn't really know him or how he was involved, so they weren't sure what to do with him. He'd driven into town and asked me out for a walk in High Park. He left his backpack in my parents' basement, and when we got back, we saw it open at the front door, a pound of weed in a vacuum-sealed bag next to it.

Why'd he even bring it in? He said it was safer in the house. Bullshit: his car was still locked. Case in point. It was a vacuum-sealed bag, too! I hadn't smoked anything. I promise! I was on probation, after all. I had to worry about piss tests, etc.

My folks were furious. My parents put together that he'd been my business partner and tried to make sure I wouldn't be seeing Chud anymore. He got through their lines of defence one more time, to meet me at a pub at Bloor and Kennedy and unassumingly push a manila envelope with twenty thousand dollars and a few grams of DMT over my way. He was sending me off with a care package. He paid for the drinks and appetizers and drove off in that flashy-ass Mercedes through affluent Bloor West Village, bass thumping some rapper saying something about pumping rock on some ghetto block.

The boom time was bust. I was on my own.

I'd be in and out of the game over the next few years, but never again at the same scale. Never again so brazenly. Never again so free.

SIX

Retrospective on 2012

We were drug buddies, first and foremost, me and the ex. We met in 2009 when she was looking for some weed and a mutual acquaintance introduced her to me; I sold her a bag of reefer, and we burned some bowls together, just talking through the night as a house party raged around us.

She was pretty ... really pretty. Tall, tanned, thin, and curvy in all the right and respective places. Brunette: she had all the physical attributes I'd been admiring in pop culture for the last few years. Immediate physical attraction.

When she arrived at my door, I was midway through a game of chess. It was a well-matched game, and it could've gone either way. I'm not sure if she acted as a muse, or if my buddy lost his focus, but soon I was wiping up his pawns, then rooks and bishops. I took his queen, and he tried to stall out for a stalemate, but I cornered him. Checkmate. I was more "with it" than usual. Normally, this guy would've cleaned my clock. Whatever the backstory, I was glad I won. It meshed well with my need to show off to a pretty girl.

"Wanna play me?"

She had a somewhat nasal voice, but it wasn't off-putting. My buddy took his cue and left. I scaled her weed and packed a bowl of mine, offering her the bong. She took it and began pulling what looked like liquid cotton through the bowl, through the water, through the bong's neck, through her lungs, and pushed it back out through her nose to hang around our heads like halos.

Shit, she could rip a bong with the best of 'em. Iron lung. Maybe that explained the nasal tone in the voice? Just perma-fucked sinuses?

—I could play again.

We set up the pieces.

"I like your walls."

It didn't seem as strange to hear back then as it would now. I was a different person, and I had different walls. They were painted electric green and covered in Sharpie doodles and quotes. I'd done a mural of a sunset over my bed, and there were poems scrawled in the spaces between the signatures of all my closest acquaintances. It would have seemed stranger to me if she hadn't liked the walls. They were objectively cool, at the time, but they looked pretty juvenile, in retrospect.

—Thanks. I think they're dope-swizzy. Do you wanna be white or black?

"Black."

That's what I would've said. There was a deeper attraction. I felt it intensely. I wondered what she felt.

She wasn't dressed to impress. Not wearing the party gear all the other girls in the house were. She was wearing sweatpants, a sweater, and moccasins. No makeup. She didn't need any of that shit. She'd just come over to buy weed and, apparently, to beat me handily at chess, which she did in fewer moves than I'd like to admit ... especially right after I'd slaughtered my buddy's lineup with such gusto. I appreciated wearing comfy clothes. It's what I do. I can't say for sure, but I assume I'd like wearing comfy clothes no matter what gender I was. I'm just a comfy-clothes person. We talked about all sorts of stuff: politics (she came from a conservative family, while mine was more liberal), music (she liked Tupac, I liked Biggie), school work (I was switching from biology to philosophy at the time, she was studying something useful), gossip (who were all those people at the party?), comfy clothing (we both wanted a pair of Uggs), etc.

"Well, it was nice meeting you. I guess, see you around."

—Yeah. Catch ya on the flip side.

She caught herself before she left. As if she'd bookmarked a thought.

"Oh, can I sign your wall?"

—Of course.

I thought she had cute handwriting. Nothing special. I don't know why I thought it was cute, but I did.

I played it cool, but I didn't want her to go. I was lonely. I was infatuated. I was forlorn. I was hopeless. She was gone. Oh well. Better luck next time ... except:

—Hey! How's it going? Remember last night?

I saw her on campus the next day, walking from one lecture hall to the next. Kismet. What a shitty opener, though. "Remember last night?" She was more sober than I was ... Oh, and she was with a friend.

"Oh, hey … hi."

She didn't seem to remember my name. Erm. What now? I opened my arms. A hug? The fuck am I doing?

She smiled at her friend, and said:

"See ya later."

Her friend left. Then she hugged me. She actually hugged me. We exchanged numbers and set up a date. This was going to be the beginning of a long and beautiful relationship, I thought.

We moved in together fairly quickly.

A good rule for a relationship is not to found it on a shared love of drugs … or any addiction, for that matter. But she was my first partner. These things have a way of spiralling, but I didn't know that at the time. We bounced bad ideas off each other, and it became very hard to lessen the intake of any given substance … especially since there was a shared supply. It gets pretty hard when you're tailoring off a drug and you see your partner ratchet up their own intake. It spurs bad juju toward the other person and fuels petty squabbles.

We introduced each other to new drugs. I discovered my love of poppers through her, reignited my love affair with tobacco, and had my first forays with cocaine. We dabbled deep in opiates together. It was clear to any objective observer that we were bad for each other.

The real issues started when she suddenly decided to stop using all of the drugs that I'd become accustomed to. She even stopped smoking weed. Good. Clearly a solid life move. This should gradually encourage me to tailor off the drugs myself, I figured, not having someone to push my exploits further and further. But she wanted me to quit everything, too, and soon.

* * *

It was shortly after my January graduation that she confronted me. Well, maybe *confronted* is just how I saw it ... let's say, she approached me with:

"This isn't working."

—Us?

I knew things weren't great. We'd been fighting. But we were salvageable. I knew that. I couldn't lose her. As unwell as I was, I knew I'd be worse off alone. I wasn't really thinking that much of what was best for her, though. Honestly, I was focusing on an ad playing on TV for P90X and thinking about how much of a loser you must be to buy into this whole "health and wellness" line. I was feelin' just dandy enough as was.

"No, not us. We're fine. I mean, not fine, that's why I'm bringing this up, but we're good ... I mean the drugs. The drugs aren't working."

I dunno about her, but I could still get high as fuck. I was pretty high already, having just sniffed twenty milligrams of OxyContin and a similar-sized line of coke. And, of course, the bong in my hand. I was confused. The drugs weren't working? What'd she mean?

"I don't want to do drugs anymore."

This brought me closer to sobriety. I felt threatened. I didn't respond, though. I didn't know how to. I noticed then that she was wearing a dress. She had lipstick on. Where was she off to?

"I don't want you to do drugs anymore, either."

This brought me closer to anger. Say what you will about me, but leave the drugs alone. They're all I had, aside from her.

—You're cutting me off?

I tried my hand at polemics, but sloppily. Even if I did harbour enough ill will against her, I was doped beyond the point of my mental faculties being on my side. I wouldn't make it long in a game of wits or logic. I had a business to think of. I was addicted to all of it. The product, the pay, the fucked-up people I met every day. She wasn't taking this from me.

"Not right away. I'm stopping now. Everything. But I need you to slow down, with the goal of stopping. You're going to die."

Then she left, in her dress and her lipstick. Very put-together. Very suddenly put-together. I should've tried offering her one last hit before she left.

I wasn't ready. I got worked up about the hypocrisy of pouring all this stuff into your body, then suddenly stopping and expecting someone else to follow suit. I can see it from her angle now, that having given up all these substances, you don't want them in your house anymore, as a temptation. But I wasn't ready to give up my habits yet.

I doubled down on the drugs. In secret. There was the added stress of no longer feeling totally welcome in my own home, coupled with having nothing to do, what with graduating in January and having no plans to leave town. I spent my days faded out. I took a lot of toilet time and always brushed the flat surfaces around our house clean of whatever powders had polluted them. I got closer to our neighbour and his biker buddies. She didn't like having bikers in our house, so that gave me a reason to spend more time next door, where I was safe to be myself. She was working and going to school full-time while I spun out. Damn nearly spun off. She didn't have time for me, and I didn't care about myself. I did feel bad, though, about my increased consumption of drugs ... especially narcotics.

I could tell she was right. I was going to die. That didn't really bother me, but the thought of her finding out I had been doing all these drugs behind her back bothered me. It wasn't that I respected her beliefs or desires or anything; I was worried that she'd find out and leave me. That was unacceptable. I'd never been left. I didn't know — or want to know — what it did to someone already predisposed to my sort of self-centred sensitivity.

* * *

"You should tell her, man."

My neighbour was a good man. Small guy. Balding. Always wearing some sort of band T-shirt, in his midforties, someone I aspired to be. He worked in acoustic engineering, so he had all sorts of cool instruments, underground band posters, and sound oddities around his house — like you'd expect to find in Anton Newcombe's. We never really got to play with them, though. We mostly just got high and watched TV. He had cute kids and he raised them right, even if he did party with bikers.

—Dude. I'm scared. What if she leaves me?

He gave me one of those "you know you know better than that" looks.

"She's not gonna leave you, mate. She loves you. You're just on different planes right now. You'll meet up at the terminal."

I liked the way he said it. I don't know whether he knew what he'd really said. Or, at least, how I interpreted it.

—Maybe you're right. But it's a leap of faith.

"Yeah, man. But you gotta have faith in life. Especially in love."

He'd gotten divorced a few years earlier. I never asked why. I trusted his wisdom.

I decided to tell her flat out. Honesty must be the best policy. She couldn't leave me if I came to her for help. I didn't like her, but I loved her, in a sense, and I just knew she couldn't be that callous. She was a better person than me.

She was taking a shower, and the bathroom was already heavy with steam and a coconut-cream shampoo smell. It was comforting. This was a good time. I could see her silhouette through the shower curtain, with the window behind her pouring in morning light.

—Hey. I … uhh … I have to tell you something.

"What is it?"

I could hear the same infectious inflection that had been there for weeks.

—I've been using drugs lately. More than you know about.

She straightened up from washing her legs. She wasn't moving. Silence for about thirty seconds, then a terse voice: "What drugs?"

—The ones I'm concerned about are coke and OxyContin.

"I can't believe you."

—I'm so sorry.

"You know what this means?"

—I need help. Please, I need help.

"I can't help you anymore."

—What do you mean?

"You're on your own."

—You're breaking up with me?

She took a moment to think.

"For now."

—What?

"I can't deal with this right now. If you can get your shit together, we can talk about us. If you can't … we can't."

I walked out of the bathroom and straight into a Baggie. Were we broken up? I didn't even know. Was this worse than being broken up? What did she want from me? Was it her or the drugs? Of course, it's her. Except, what was I doing with the Baggie? Java, who generally followed me everywhere, looked up at me like she knew what was going on better than I did.

I don't know what I really expected. I vaguely hoped for compassion. Maybe, addict to addict, she'd understand. Maybe honesty really was the best policy, like everyone says.

Nope.

That was the last day of our relationship.

SEVEN

2017

When I'm deep in mental illness, I feel infectious. I mean, I guess I am infectious, even if it's just my mood. But mood disorders aren't clinically contagious … not like the plague. More like old age. You can feel it in the air, and it might affect you … but can you catch depression? It feels like it when I'm depressed. Like, don't come next to me unless you're ready to be unhealthy.

When I'm empty, I feel like a black hole. As though the happy, healthy people who touch me will be taken in and never recover. I personalize anything that enters my mind. It's almost impossible to remember that everyone's on their own circular (or, for some, elliptical) orbit of some celestial body; everybody makes choices every moment of every day that affect absolutely everything in their own lives and, to lesser and lesser concentric extents, the lives of the orbiting objects around and among them.

When I'm sick, society's psychic impact tells me to withdraw, for the benefit of the herd. This mode of thinking is beyond a simple school of thought; it's a hard-wired instinct. It's billions of years of trial and error we mistakenly call evolution.

Needless to say, I feel sick more than most of the time. Whether that sickness is up or down or side to side, though, the rule remains the same — I withdraw, for the benefit of the herd. I know it's the worst thing I could do.

When I'm sick, I need parties more than most, but it's an involuntary drive that pushes me, from the inside out, to leave other people well enough alone. This omnipresent thought is made worse when, in rare moments of lucidity and consideration of others, I discover that a friend or family member has fallen grievously ill, and I draw lines of responsibility back to my own actions. It may be selfish to think that I'm the one to blame for a friend's suicide, or for my mother's sudden psychotic breakdown last year, but it feels like a selfless sort of selfishness. At least, to me it does.

EIGHT

Retrospective on 2008

A central theme to my university time was a reckless disregard for my own well-being and future. And it wasn't just me. It was all of us. Well, all the kids I got to know, at least. I could fill this book, and several others, with story after story, each stranger and more sensational than the last, just about our daily life. Here's an example of one particular day that stands out in memory.

So, 2C-B is recreationally active at around ten milligrams or so. I had a chemistry midterm later on, and I'd already dropped a weak tab of acid (about one hundred micrograms), so I didn't want to get too fucked up. Little did we know that we'd been provided with misinformation about the next drop in our cocktail. Our capsules each held one hundred milligrams — the dose recommended by the dealer ... So we trusted him and popped our capsules.

I've never done an appropriate amount of 2C-B. I know this now. I've done it a few times, but it was never quite something I could get into. I did a full hundred milligrams, maybe ten times or so the recommended dose, several times. I hear it's a simply lovely drug and excellent for therapy and microdosing, but in my experience, at least, it's very fucking weird. It had been marketed "like MDMA when you move, like LSD when you sit down." That sounded cool to me.

My roommate, Teddy, who was my business partner at the time, had some connections from his hometown coming down later in the day, before my midterm (which, as you may have guessed, I wasn't studying for). Teddy was, as the name suggests, a big cuddle puddle. He was about my size, but he seemed bigger. He was exuberant. Friendly to the tune of *Barney & Friends*, just less overtly creepy. He always wore something cozy, but invariably designer made. Leisure was his life. He loved weed. Occasionally, he'd try something fucked up that I'd give him ... but aside from that, he was a ganja chimney garbed in trendy sweaters, sweatpants, and big fuzzy boots. Together we stoked climbing cholesterol counts and the diet that would eventually culminate in my developing gout and prediabetes before thirty. Everything Teddy did was about feeling good. School work? Not interested. Real business? Not interested. Getting high and playing N64? "Tell me more."

Teddy's friends came to our room and got to work showing us their wares. We responded in kind, seeing if we could trade anything, and we all pulled out cash to settle the odd numbers.

We were getting to a place of proper nonsensicality, and we were smoking blunts with the window closed, for some reason. Likely stupidity. Five of us sat in the small room, spread over two parallel beds and a desk pushed up against the wall, perpendicular to the beds and across the room from the door — about ten or twelve feet long, ten or so feet wide. It was cramped.

The room stank like yogurt. Not fresh yogurt. More like poorly curdled, flavoured kefir. The smell could've been coming from anywhere, but it sliced through the cess smoke like the sound of a sitar through silence, or like a scimitar through that same sitar. It was sharp. I suppose a prime suspect would've been the small, neon-green acrylic bong we called "Puff," which we'd filled with chocolate milk a few weeks before (purely to see what smoking through chocolate milk does) and just never cleaned out. It could've been Teddy's socks ... I think the big dude might have caught a foot fungus from the dormitory showers.

Teddy and I had been responsible for the upkeep of this room for the past six months, and it felt like a leper colony. We were at a point where we chilled in other people's rooms. But when it came to business, it was safer done in room four-twenty. (That's right. The university chose it for us.)

We didn't even realize the door was ajar. My residence assistant walked in. She took a quick look around the room. Shit.

"Guys, can someone explain what's going on?"

I think she got a pretty reasonable sense of what was going on.

Silence, then a golden ticket.

"Mary? Is that you?"

"Yeah. Who are you?"

"It's [some guy]."

"Oh my God! How are you doing? I haven't seen you since, like, grade nine. What are you up to these days?"

He looked at the floor, where a half pound was still sitting on a scale.

"Right. Well, listen up, guys. I'm not going to report this, but I don't condone it or want to see it again. All right?"

Sounded fair to me. We all nodded (with no intention of following through) like chastised lion cubs. She turned around and walked away. Teddy jumped up to close the door, lock it, and open the window, turning on the fan and spraying Febreze. He was more "on it" than I was. I was full in the grips of ten times as much 2C-B as was recommended. I felt like Syd Barrett on a bad day.

We somehow completed the transactions and the guys left. We both lay down with headphones on, hoping to ride it all out. I should've looked up how long 2C-B lasted before taking it, especially considering I had a chemistry midterm in five hours. "Killer Chem," they called it. The average for the midterm the year before was 48 percent. I should've studied.

I pulled up the blankets and noticed how strangely synthetic the drug was. The visuals were all urban graffiti motifs, and I felt like I was on the subway, for some reason. I focused on a wormhole in the cupboard where no visible light reached. It was a cave. There was something in that cave. Something dark. It looked like a machine elf and observed me like the Morrigan. Where was this all going? I watched that cave until my alarm went off. Exam time! Fuck, still kinda really tripping.

I got to the exam. Good start. I was on time. I wrote the exam. That was a little more intense than finding the exam hall, but I finished it at least. I would later find out I'd actually passed. Hey, that's all I'd gone to do. I'd done all right, too. Not, like, the best I could do ... but I made it through. The numbers and patterns and molecular shapes just sort of made sense to me. New formulas formulated deep in my, ironically, chemically reconstructed cerebrum. It all fell into line. I'm terrible at mental math, but something seems to have clicked after the introduction of mass amounts of psychedelics. Maybe there was something to the Dock Ellis story, or to Crick coming up with the helical structure of DNA while on acid ...

Maybe Rosalind Franklin knows.

When I got back to our room, Teddy was ripping a bowl through Puff. He coughed pretty hard, despite having packed ultra-smooth cannabis. Maybe we should've refreshed the chocolate milk more often. I sat down on my bed and watched him hold in some vomit.

—Dude. That was fucking close this morning.

He swallowed whatever was in his mouth.

"What was?"

—Mary walking in. Dude ... if we didn't have [some guy], we'd be ... somewhere else.

"Like, expelled?"

—No, dude, we'd be in jail.

"Oh, yeah. True."

He wasn't even fazed. Amazing.

—You wanna celebrate?

"Celebrate what?"

—Never mind. Oh, I went to the Killer Chem exam, man! I even finished it. I was thinking you might be down to bomb some hills?

"Hell yeah, dude. Sounds dope. I wanna do the one down Main Street."

I didn't know if my longboard could handle going that fast.

—That's suicide.

"You down?"

—Like a suicidal clown, man. I know how to make it even better.

Reaching into my bottom drawer, I pulled out some cough syrup. Promethazine and codeine were the main things we were looking for from this bottle. Though, it did taste good. I grabbed a Sprite, some Jolly Ranchers, and two kegger cups and got to mixing.

—Cheers, man!

"Bottoms up."

It tasted significantly better than some other types of cough syrup I'd drunk.

We conscripted a few of our longboard crew to come with, but none of them were as fucked as we were. One of them brought his car so he could track our speed going down the hill.

My buddy yelled at me from the car window:

"You're going eighty kilometres an hour, man!"

I had a "mortality moment." I was on two psychedelics … acid and a massive dose of 2C-B. I was getting slurry and sloppy from the cough syrup, and all the weed and beers I didn't even really count.

—Don't say any more. I wanna stop!

"You gotta ride it, man."

Ahhh fuuuck. I became hyperconscious of every move I made, every crack in the asphalt, all the cars around me I was careening through. Dodging fucking manholes like land mines.

Eventually the road levelled out, and I put down my foot to skid to a stop. I wanted to do it again.

As I said, a reckless disregard for my well-being. I could've died. Fuck. I was eighteen. I wasn't wearing a helmet. I was in a wolf T-shirt, shorts, and sandals. Imagine the corpse.

When we got home, we were pretty frazzled by the day; though, to be fair, this was the usual. Teddy started getting the mini-packets ready for a microwave soup. Some sort of shitty ramen. I got into a shirt and underwear and threw on a nature documentary. The door played a drumroll.

"What's up, guys?"

It was Fred. Pretty-boy Fred. Fred was always to the point. He brought business, and he sometimes did business with us. He was business. Fred had a pint in his hand. A pint that brought the smell of cheap rum into the room, mixing with the yogurt odours. Teddy started heading down the hall to the common room, where the microwave was, also in boxers and a T-shirt.

"Just makin' some soup, Fred. What's up?"

"I brought people who want weed."

—How much?

Fred came into the room so I could see the visitors he'd brought us. They stayed firmly outside the doorway, in the hall. It was two guys with a hookah. In-con-fucking-spicuous. They looked younger than we did, and we were eighteen. They were just two kids looking to get high in a way only the practically innocent could — out in the open with a fucking hookah. One of them was wearing torn jeans and a Donovan shirt; the other was in brown corduroy pants with a high-school rowing team jersey. Where did Fred find these kids? They were looking at our room like they were watching a beheading video. What a mess we must've made.

"Just like, a nickel?"

The guy's voice quavered. He was scared.

I looked at Fred. He looked at them like he could kill them. His brow furrowed in a way I recognized. For such a good-looking guy, he sure could crank up the scary vibes. His family was connected. Not that it matters. But he'd been around heavy shit going down as far back as he could remember. He always struck me as looking and acting like the demon from the end of the original *Fantasia* film. You know, "Night on Bald Mountain," evil. He also cast a striking resemblance to the Jim Morrison poster we'd plastered on our wall, "American Poet." Like both Morrison and the demon, Fred played with people. He was good at it. He prided himself on it. And I could tell he felt played by these guys. They'd asked him for weed. And everyone knew Fred didn't fuck around with small-time shit. Five dollars is not a deal worth making when you have thousands of illicit dollars sitting in a hollowed-out stolen library book. Not that the library book being stolen would probably add much to the primary charges.

"Are you fucking kidding me?"

—Fred, it's all right. They're here already. I'll do it.

We shot the shit for a bit, largely ignoring the other kids. I told him about my day, and I noticed them tense up a bit. I got a little rush out of the idea of my daily life being intimidating. Then I focused back on Fred. Fred dealt on a level almost as large as we did, but he primarily sold ketamine. He did a lot of it, too. Sometimes seven or so grams a day. A reasonable dose is, say, fifty milligrams. He did Hollywoods — lines long enough that one day his nasal cavity collapsed and he needed surgery. He said the sky was always purple static. All he'd do was snort ketamine, play Hendrix-level guitar (but he'd prefer being compared to Paco de Lucía), work out, and run calculus and geometry programs on his computer, producing beautiful mathematical patterns. A gifted mind gone adrift.

Teddy was back by the time I'd pulled out my smallest bag of weed, so as not to give away to these strangers the scale of our operations.

"Where'd the hookah dudes go?"

Neither Fred nor I had noticed that our visitors had quietly slipped away while we were talking, and I was preparing to sell the smallest increment of weed I'd sold in years. Teddy came in and started eating soup and getting ready for bed. He was always ready for bed. Beddy-bye Teddy.

"I'm gonna fuck them up."

—Man, leave it, Fred. They got scared off.

"Oh shit! You scared off the hookah guys?" Teddy chirped with amusement.

He was already spilling ramen noodles and desiccated vegetable flakes on his Spider-Man comforter. Fucking slob. His half of the room was always dirty laundry and biohazards made of last month's meals exposed to lingering ganja smoke.

—I think our lifestyle disagrees with them. Man, I'm going to bed. Catch you later, Fred.

Fred took a pissed-off look down the hallway. He nodded at us and strode off with his pint of rum.

I thought little more of it and was drifting down, down, down into the down of my pillow, watching a shark gnash at seabirds on the computer screen, sliding into blackness as my eyelids went slack. Then a rap on the door.

—Who's that?

"Fred."

I opened the door. There was blood on Fred's right hand and two thirds of the pint of rum left in his glass.

—What's up, dude?

"I knocked out those fuckwits. I saw them smoking that fucking hookah on the hill, and I just beat the shit outta them. What do they do that for? Make me interrupt my friends while they're getting ready for bed, just for five bucks of weed? Then they run out before they even buy anything? What the fuck, man?"

Teddy chimed in: "Dude, it's really not a big deal. Thanks for punching people for us, though."

"But they interrupted your soup, man …"

He wandered off back down the hall to his ketamine, calculus, geometry, and flamenco guitar, which echoed his frustrations back to us dreamily in what seemed like the syncopated steps of a delightfully dressed dancer leading me to sleep.

Yeah. A "normal" sort of day. If you'd asked me at the time if anything out of the ordinary had happened, I'd have probably started off by telling you what I had for breakfast. A quesadilla. Commonly crazy.

NINE

Retrospective on 2011

I've met some strange kids in this industry. Most of them are eerily endearing, in their own ways, with contrarians and generally rowdy rule breakers being attracted to the business — like orphans to extremism. It has something verboten about it. But, now and then, you hit a truly odd duck.

I'll call this guy Leprechaun 'cause he's Irish, and they caught him and his pot of gold. He kind of reminded me of Soulless, just a bit more rugged. Unpolished. He wasn't as smooth of a criminal. Sure, Soulless bumped Biggie out of a shitbox car and had his driver in tow at all times — but he didn't look like a big spender. No doubt, he had the funds for a flashier life; he just saved and invested it. He was quiet. Leprechaun was loud. He flouted his earnings. He caught the attention of cops.

Nothing remarkable about Leprechaun's appearance. Dirty-blond hair. Not thin, not fat. A little shorter than me but a little taller than most. He was wearing a Leafs jersey and a Leafs hat. There wasn't even a game that night. He wasn't even really *weird*, exactly. It's just, sort of like a Leprechaun, when you looked a little closer, he wasn't really there. As in, in a human way. I never felt like I was in the room with a person when we'd visit Leprechaun. He felt more like a predator in a zoo. Like a bear or a tiger. Biding his time and watching the zookeepers to see which one would slip up first, and where. Oh sure, he might roll over in return for a raw steak, but he was still akin to a wild animal at the end of the day. And forgetting such was done at your own peril.

He was the older brother of a girl Chud was involved with, which gave us an in to yet another high-grade, high-level distributor. Except all Leprechaun sold was reefer-related materials and coke. Yet we'd drive into the city to see him: it was that good and the price was that right. He did bulk buys only.

Chud had a story about being in the passenger seat, driving down the highway with Leprechaun when the latter's business phone rang. Considering it was his business phone, it was a high-end piece of hardware. Dude splurged big on everything. Answering it, while driving, with ki's in the boot, he got visibly upset. Something wasn't going right.

"What the fuck do you mean you can't do it? Know what you really can't do? Fuck me! I fuck back, motherfucker!"

Then, according to Chud, Leprechaun didn't hang up on the guy so much as throw his phone out the window, directly into the windshield of another car, which spun out and got rammed by a series of other cars. Leprechaun didn't give a fuck.

"Hey, look! Open roads, man. Always a silver fuckin' lining."

Whenever we rolled up to visit him, we'd park a few blocks away and walk up to his lakefront condo, then go to his classic coke-lord penthouse. It had everything aside from a guy in a Speedo tossing cherry bombs. We parked a few blocks away not because his guest parking was being watched — but because he already had three luxury sports cars in the garage.

The centrepiece of the condo, the focal point, was between two doorways that led onto the huge balcony, the sort of spot where usually you'd see a TV. There sat a massive saltwater aquarium, complete with colourful tropical fish, a little metal dude in the deep-sea diver outfit ... all of it — especially, for the purposes of this story, a tiny little sucker fish, nondescript in appearance, dwarfed by the graceful rainbow-stylized angel-fish gliding past. The sucker fish was feeding off the shit and leftover scraps of the others. Leprechaun walked up to the tank and pointed at the bottom-feeder:

"See this little shit-eater here? That's Ed. Know why I named him Ed?"

I looked at another dude sitting on the couch. A dude who didn't give off the vibes of a caged predator. He needed a trip to the dentist. And probably an orthodontist. And basically every other health service available. His hair was falling out. His fingernails were dirty, broken, or missing. His skin was damn near translucent ... lots of yellow and blue, blending in a way that made me feel green. Both sick and naive to what was going on. Who was this guy? He didn't fit this luxury con-do. He did have very new and clean clothes, for some reason, but they were very cheap. Sweatpants and a shirt. All white. I thought there should be more stains, in keeping with the rest of him, but his attire was tip-top. The way he sat, the way his sweatpants draped over his crotch, I could tell that all of him was flaccid. He seemed removed from the rest of us, but he wasn't, at least not physically. It was like he was in a boring trance. He seemed as dull as *The Stranger*. Mundane, blasé, unmindfully nihilistic.

Leprechaun repeated his question: "Hey. Know why I named him Ed?"

This was directed past me, to the guy on the couch.

"Yessir."

The sloppy guy just sort of gurgled out his answer. Something *très étrange* was going on, and I felt uncomfortable.

I looked back at the sucker fish, and it darted out of the way of a shadow cast by a larger fish. The fish I'd normally notice first. The sloppy guy wasn't any more forthcoming, so Leprechaun enlightened Chud and me.

"That little shit-eating fish is Ed. Ed's *there* to remind Eddie *here* what he is. He's a shit-eater. He lives off me. He's a parasite. Aren't you, Ed?"

"Yessir."

He sounded so defeated. At least he had a name now.

Again, Leprechaun spoke, but this time there was an edge. He snapped at Eddie: "Hey, Ed. Be a good shit-eater and get us some chocolate milk."

Leprechaun extended his hand, holding a ten-dollar bill, and waited for Eddie to take it. Eddie looked hungry. Eddie looked thirsty.

"Can I —"

Leprechaun shut that bright idea down with an eyebrow. He grunted: "You'll get what you get. Got it?"

Eddie couldn't have looked more downcast if he were trying for the cast of *Les Misérables*.

"Yessir."

Eddie took the ten and went downstairs to the convenience store to get us some chocolate milk. Once he'd gone,
Leprechaun pulled out a bag with what looked like a bunch
of small, uncut gemstones in it ... I knew better, though. He
took his time selecting one the right size and put it on the table.
I knew better than to ask questions. If I needed to know, it'd
come up.

"Ed's useful, but you gotta keep him down. I give him
clothes, to keep my place fresh, 'cause he fuckin' stinks, and
I give him some food, but I don't give him jackshit else. You
can't let him realize the other fish depend on him. It only works
while Ed believes he's a shit-eater. Above all, you need two
things — not to forget that Ed's seen all your dirt, and to keep
Ed dependent on you. You guys should get an Ed."

He looked gently down at the pebble on the table.

"I hate cooking rocks. It's so much work, and it's just for
fuckin' Ed. I wish I could switch him to meth or something."

Eddie came back with chocolate milk. He put it down on
the table and moved in on his crack allowance. Leprechaun
wasn't done, though.

"We want glasses, Ed. Pour them."

I thought I'd seen everything at that point, but I'd never
watched a crackhead place a rock on a table, hands shivering,
to pour three grown men their cups of chocolate milk, without
spilling, then stand back up to wait for dismissal.

If I were Eddie, I would've fucking flipped. (I have to assume. I don't know. I don't think I've ever done crack, so I'm
totally unqualified to predict a crackhead's movements.) At
least, if it were me as *me*, I would've cracked wayyy before that
point and just fuckin' pulverized Leprechaun, Nazino Island
style. Honestly ... that was such a prick move! And Eddie

didn't even let a moment of blood lust cross his face. Just regret that he hadn't acted appropriately. This person was broken.

"There you go, Ed. That wasn't so hard. Now go and blow your fuckin' brains out on that, you retarded shit-eating fish fuck."

Eddie took it in stride — got his crack and hightailed it to the balcony, where his pipe was waiting. He wasn't allowed to smoke inside.

Leprechaun lit a cigarette and offered one to each of us.

Sure.

"Good system I've got with Ed, eh?"

I was speechless, thinking hard on what to say. Leprechaun had asked us a question outright. He wanted an answer. We needed an answer. Chud, too, had remained essentially speechless for most of this but apparently had the gusto to ask the question I'd been trying so delicately to formulate into a sentence:

"So ... Ed's like ... your slave?"

Leprechaun pinched his lips together in thought, and I anticipated a reproach for the direct approach Chud was taking. Then his face relaxed. He looked at peace. Like a well-fed tiger smiling over his shoulder as he strides out of the zoo into the sunset.

"Crack slave. Yeah."

On the way back, after the deal, with the product in the trunk and Leprechaun a safe hundred or so kilometres away, I asked Chud:

—So that Eddie thing ...

Immediate response: "THAT WAS SO FUCKIN' FUCKED! Oh my God, man. Jesus! Holy fucking shit that was weird!"

I rolled and licked and lit a spliff, lowering my window just enough to ash outside without freezing my fingers in the winter air. We were often fairly indiscreet about basically hotboxing a car on the highway. Chud had gone to a police fundraiser some years before and gotten the cheapest thing there: a sticker displaying the logo of our university town's police force. Like, a two-dollar sticker. What a fuckin' investment, though. It got us out of trouble a ridiculous number of times. Twenty pounds in the trunk? Not a problem. Cops would pull us over, and we'd light a cigarette each to cover the *Reefer Madness* smell, then we'd just act normal. We had nothing to hide. We were just two clean-cut(ish) white dudes in our twenties out for a drive. Just getting stuff done.

Chud always had a cover story: "Hey there, bud! My uncle's on the force out in Hamilton, and I've always thought of going that way myself. Just trying to support the cause, eh?" He had the wickedest grin.

And some cops like white boys: "You don't say? Well, you two take it easy out here tonight, eh? Noticed you were going a bit over the limit. Gotta watch out for the black ice."

Chud would respond with something like, "Will do, my good man. You too. Thank you for your service."

And off we'd go. Back on our way to Hell.

We got into the philosophical ramifications of the "Eddie-ness" of it all, not to mention the logistics ... making sure he doesn't flip, etc.

"Do you think he has something on Eddie? Like, dirt? Or, like, is he threatening Eddie's family or something?"

—I think it's just crack, man. Crack's fucked.

"You think Ed couldn't kick it? He didn't look happy with life. Like, c'mon man, just quit, if that's all it is."

—That might be all it is on the surface. But what about the rest of it? Like, why's he on crack to begin with?

"Hah. 'Cause his fuckin' life fuckin' sucks."

I want to be more serious about this. I don't know why.

—I don't think happy people start smoking crack, dude. I think it's the last-ditch effort of the damned to claw back a momentary trace of dopamine. It's a last resort. Like, you saw him … he's a slave. He can't be happy. Not in any way. I doubt even the crack makes him happy. It's just a Band-Aid solution. Patching up the crack, y'know?

Chud smiles.

"Patching up the crack. I like that … Do you think he'd ever flip on [Leprechaun]?"

—I dunno, man. Ask Haiti. Ask Spartacus.

Chud focused on the road. It was snowing. There were about two or three minutes of radio silence between us while he seemed to be thinking hard about something.

"Smart of [Leprechaun] to dress him all in white."

—Why's that?

"He can't escape."

I thought about it. That was true. It was a fail-safe Leprechaun had implemented. He used the cover "to keep my place fresh" when really it was meant to make Eddie stand out. Skid row–looking guy wearing all white. Those clothes would stain up quickly if he got loose. That would make him stand out even more. He wouldn't be able to hide. Especially not with all the ears and eyes around the city that Leprechaun had paid for.

—Man. I feel kinda fucked up.

"Me too, man. Me too."

—Why do you feel fucked up?

"This spliff, man ... You?"

—Same.

Chud turned to me with a truly sick grin:

"Still. Hard to argue with results. I mean ... chocolate milk on tap? What a fuckin' dream."

A few years later I heard Leprechaun had been scooped on attempted murder. I wondered if it had anything to do with Eddie.

No. Eddie wasn't that important.

TEN

Retrospective on 2008

Down by the banks of the river, you could usually find a quiet, dark place to burn a doobie in privacy or have a conversation, or both. Whatever. I wasn't alone, but I wasn't particularly keen on conversation. Skittles was excited, as usual, to be hanging out with me. I was scratching my growing beard and looking out over the reeds, listening to the trickle of water as it meandered over rocks in a shallow spot. I was thinking of just letting my beard go. I hadn't tried it yet. My sister made sure I was shaving as soon as I had peach fuzz. She wasn't going to let me be one of those guys. But now it was coming in dark. I hadn't shaved in a few weeks, and it was long enough to pretend to stroke and really need to scratch. People tell me my beard has every colour of hair in it: red, brown, blond, black, grey, and white. White hairs at eighteen. Shit.

"Hey, hey, there's a spot near my parents' house. I wanna take you."

—Why?

"It's, uh, it's a spot under a bridge. Well, not under it — it's, uh, like in it. You're, like, hundreds of feet up, and you can climb through a fence and into this nook place. It's cool. It's got an awesome view of the city. It's really cool. It's a great place to hang out and smoke a joint."

—Yeah.

"I like bridges. They're so representative. Like, they're bridges. To all sorts of things! Isn't that cool?"

—There are a few cool bridges, I guess.

"Ha ha ha. This is a cool bridge. We should go sometime, whenever we go back to Toronto, we could hang out."

—I'm afraid of heights.

"Oh. Why? I didn't think you were afraid of anything. It's cool."

—I always feel like there's a tube sticking out of my head and it's sucking me over the edge. I have to be a few feet away from the drop if it's more than about thirty feet. I feel like it's an inevitability that I'm going over the side.

"Whoa. That's trippy, man."

—Wouldn't wanna trip, would I now?

He smiled a smile so wide it could crack its own sides.

"Have you ever tried one of these?"

It was impossible to tell in the dark what he was gesticulating at, but he was down by the reeds, where all the grimy shit was.

—What is it?

"It looks like a jimson weed pod."

—Here, pass it over.

I needed to get a hold of it before he'd shoved it all in his gob. And knowing Skittles, he'd probably eat every bit of it if I said it could get you high. Being as tiny as he was, too ... fuck. No clue what would happen to him.

I've never had the stuff before. Nor, probably, will I. I know it has a long history of use around the world, for many purposes from analgesic to shamanistic, but there are always going to be certain plants and chemicals I just don't want to try. Even I'm scared of them. Ibogaine comes to mind. Jimson weed is one of those.

Jimson weed, or *Datura stramonium*, contains all sorts of horrifying shit. Not the least of worth mentioning is scopolamine. The dangerous chemicals are spread throughout the plant, the leaves, the shoots, and the roots, but it's the seeds you really gotta watch out for. It's sometimes used "recreationally" (or given the effects, positively forcefully-spiritually) or medicinally, but it should always be administered by trained — I dunno — administering agents. The drug even gets a disclaimer in *Fear and Loathing*, which should indicate the possible absurdity with which I was faced. Dosing is particularly precarious, even if I knew the relative alkaloid levels present in this particular pod.

I may not have tried these substances, but I've studied them as best I can. I want to be a well-rounded psychonaut, after all.

Skittles handed me the pod. It was jimson weed, clear as day. Spiky case, tons of tiny, dark seeds. Right biome. It looked like an evil poppy. I chucked it out into the water. It plopped gently out of our possible evening plans. I stood up and once again towered over Skittles. I always seemed to tower over

Skittles. Everyone did. It was time to go back to the dorm. I
didn't wanna be around this guy anymore. I was bored.

—Nah, that's not jimson weed. Don't do that shit, though.
Stuff like that can kill you.

"Cool, man. Wouldn't it be fucked to die while you're
tripping?"

The sky started pissing a fine mist over us. It was cold.
The wind picked up and slipped through my light jacket and
sweater and into my bones. Into my soul. Or whatever you call
the spectral anomaly that goes in that hole. I sped up my walk.
He began jogging to keep up.

—I guess it depends on what you're tripping on.

"Ha ha ha. You know how people say you can trip on life?
Do you think you can trip on death?"

I didn't know what he meant.

—I think you can trip while dying. But I think the trip
ends when there's no tripper left.

He looked consternated.

"Dude, I never wanna stop tripping."

We were in sight of the residence building. I wouldn't have
to deal with his insipid insights for long. I could just say I was
tired and close my door. From there, only Teddy had the ability
to bother me. I was in a bad mood, for some reason, but I was
still cognizant enough to take care of business:

—Don't worry. I'm here.

ELEVEN

2015

In between the loop-de-loops on this radical roller coaster of bipolar proportions, there's a series of moments of lucidity, where the G-forces keep you glued to the seat for a second and you're looking the world straight on and wayyy heavy. In these nanofractal fractions of familiarity, I get bored easily. Call it the ADHD, but maybe it's more basic than that — I'm used to the trip now, and being sober makes me feel unnatural: I've adapted to distracting abstractions.

I'm bored *now*, having taken a short respite from mind-altering substances in the past few days. I'm also mildly depressed, after having spent the day at MarineLand with my new female friend's family. "Keeper." I mentioned her before, in passing. It's not her or the family that has me down … it was the park. I've always been an animal person.

With pride in myself for having gone a whole weekend without even weed, I make a pipe out of tinfoil wrapped around a Bic pen. Discretion is the name of the game now that I'm living back at home with the oldies — even if this method isn't particularly healthy. They know I smoke weed — I mean, I have a doctor's note — but they don't know how much. And they're not particularly fond of it being in their house.

I fill the tinfoil tube with some of the fresh Neville's Haze I picked up from the dispensary earlier, sneak halfway down the ravine out back of my folks' place, and burn the whole bowl in one excited breath while looking out over the canopy surrounding the pond behind their house. I bet some teenagers are down there, tripping under the trees the way I used to. The way I still do, sometimes.

I've been living with my parents since I got back from my time at university, back in 2012. Keeper has her own place, so I spend quite a bit of time in her bachelor pad at "Young and Eligible," but my base of operations is still the bedroom I moved into when I was eight, when we moved back to Canada from our overseas odyssey. Yeah, it feels like a step back, but Keeper and I are planning on getting an apartment soon. Something in the neighbourhood. Not too far from my parents, or High Park. Or Java.

My folks' house is right by the park. Like, RIGHT by the park. Their street is adjacent to Grenadier Pond, around which I perambulate with my pup on the regular. It's my meditation. Living here has its perks … but there's a certain set of limits around how "me" I can be here. Getting out with Keeper ought to be a nice change of pace.

Back at the top of the steps, I'm heartily flushed and breaking out in a sweat. Neville's Haze ... pure sativa. Not a good medication for when you're already usually hearing things.

I glaze past the paintings on the wall and don't notice them as distinct works of art; rather, the continuity of my experience was, in itself, art. I reach the top of the carpeted stairway and stumble to the side of my bed, crumpling into the folds, merging with them as intimately as most marriages can get. My laptop opens of its own accord and immerses me in a BBC vision of *Planet Earth* — which I feel very little inherent attachment to (gravitationally or otherwise) at the moment.

I think of Keeper and want to write something for her. She deserves that much for dealing with me this last year. I fumble in the drawer of my bedside table and fail to find a notebook, then realize my laptop does more than just entertain me when I'm tripping out — it can be used *as a tool for good.*

I start clacking on the keyboard. What is this thing gonna be? Maybe I'll write a story about her. Or a poem! She loves sonnets. She studied English, unlike me. I only ever took one English course in university and it was introductory English for science and math kids. Minimal literary education. But I do have an interest, and zeal — and that's most of writing, right? OK ... let's do this thing. Iambic pentameter. Hazy stream of consciousness, do your thing:

PLANET MANIA

*Instructions for reading are as
follows:

1. Say "STOP" all old timey like
   you were on a thingy majig from

way-back-whenever, whenever you see
one of these things
    '/'

*That's it so far.

"Gems of genius left by former generations sit hidden in the rhythm given
rise to by eternal cycles of the sun."
—Me.

Writing is like riding a train where you
    decide when to jump/ off topic.
We should desalinate the planet with
    mangrove plantations and/ I want a pet
    octopus. We're all in this together,
        this/ life.
Like, seriously, Sir-for-FUCK'S-SAKES-/
David Attenborough/
it's "shrimp," not "shrimps."

    Babe, I love you so much./
Wasn't that turtle in *Finding Nemo*?/

I wanna get back to the beginning and
    retrace the trip
but I just keep spinning and screaming
    and singing and spinning and/
        skip-skip//
SPINNING SHAHSHAHAHhabajzhznajshahaha
    hahahHHaahbAha!!!@@!!!1!!?!*9!!1*!!/

That bird is huge. Certain systems will
    recycle in symbiotic security./
        Stop alliterating, my Love!/ I love
        you, babe :)/

Hahahahaha, "Sailfish live high-octane
    lives."/

Seriously though, Attenborough, dude,
you're awesome./

MarineLand was a beautiful trajedy today./
Did I misspell 'tragedy'?/

Babe, I gotta poo. I haven't gone in days./
I'm pooing.

(ii)

There were lots of deer pellets in the
park and/ the deer(s?) were moulting,
or whatever/ the word is where their
antlers come off in stringy bits/ of
blood-soaked sinew and they fight and
fuck and/ keep beating each other up.
I don't even know who was who/ or what
was what/ or something. Fuck,/ my reflection is fucked.

Fuck, and/ there was a bloated,
yellowish beluga/ being all buoyant
and shit and sideways and stuff./ I
should get out of the bathroom.

(iii)

Where did this weed come from
originally?

(iv)

*Commence episode 2 after escape outside
for another bowl.*

"Seasonal Forests." I can dig it./

"Trees — surely among the most magnificent of living things."

David-FUCKIN'-Attenborough, people!

(v)

Seriously,/ we could solve all types
of serious issues with a bit of/
ingenuity. Like the fish farm in
Eritrea before the civil war.

I got an award for marine biology in
high school.

(vi)

Suck the salt out of seawater so you
can irrigate deserts with fish shit.
Make your own sustainable ecosystems.
Pave the streets with solar panels.
Keep bees. Compost. Bike to work on
power generators.

Choose online banking./

(vii)

I should probs just conquer the world
for its own/ good.

(viii)

JKS!!

P.S. (ix)

The animals in that enchanted forest
are all so small because humans lived
there and hunted it empty then left
their pets. Duh.

(x)

Nine is an (in?)auspicious number.

* * *

What in the fuck is this? Sure, it mentions Keeper, but it's hardly for her. This doesn't seem to be a story ... it's definitely not a sonnet. Is it even a poem? Or is it the incoherent "something" produced by a maniac you just sort of let babble on? Can this shit even be edited, or should I just toss it?

TWELVE
2017

Whenever I meet a new psychiatrist or psychologist or social worker or occupational therapist or emergency nurse or group facilitator, they make an assumption that I come from a troubled home. Then they meet my parents, who usually accompany me to the hospital (since my memory isn't what it used to be, and I often need a second set of ears). I was definitely born into the one percent. Maybe even the one percent of the one percent, globally, at least.

My mom spent most of my childhood as a functionally tipsy housewife, then returned to the workforce as a tax collector in my early teens. My mom made the bread a normal family would depend on, but my dad made the bacon, freeing up my mom's salary, and subsequent early pension, for trips abroad, extravagant house parties, absurd Christmas present piles, and a guaranteed education for as far as I wanted to take it. Dad's in the senior echelons of the executive class of the Canadian-based, internationally reaching banking system, and his career trajectory is the wet dream of every MBA or CA student in the world. His various postings took our family on an international tour of the planet's tax havens.

My sister was born in Australia three and a half years before me. I was born during a brief stopover back in Toronto before we moved to Barbados a year later, then it was on to the Isle of Jersey (Jersey of *Forbes* fame — ye *Olde* Bailiwick of Jersey). My childhood best friend's father was one of the wealthiest men in Britain at the time. I was exposed, from as soon as I could recognize it, to unnecessary levels of comfort and accommodation.

We aren't, like, the Eaton or Rothschild or Kennedy families or anything. We weren't like the kids I went to school with. The old aristocracy of Europe escaping estate taxes. Titled classmates. Viscount Charles or Marquis Pierce. My sister and I were "Master" and "Miss" [last name]. But my sister's more fortunate friends, on paper at least, were "Lady Such-and-such." But those old families … watch out for the generational trauma. Not to mention the inbreeding. Everyone's mansion highlighted a massive family tree that inevitably began with Charlemagne, and everyone was related in some way or other.

We're lower upper class. I used to think we were middle class, then I met middle-class kids in Canada and was told otherwise. My dad was in Jersey to work for the ultrarich, managing their legacy fortunes, but I was spoiled by proximity. Poorest kid in the school, apart from my sister, I got by on my exotic-ness (having a five-year-old's Bajan accent) until it developed into an aristocratic parody: poshness from the resident peasant.

My sister and I were close friends during our world tour; she was usually the only other kid to play with, and she was a good, gentle sister. I'd sleep under her bed, hiding from the monsters under mine and keeping those under hers at bay. She'd dress me up and put makeup on me. I was the little sister she'd always wanted.

And to boot, my folks are simply lovely people. Totally self-made and accepting of almost everyone. As liberal as they could possibly be, given the restrictions of the circles we travelled in.

You might be wondering now, if this guy comes from money, why'd he do all this dumb shit? There are a number of factors. My parents were always very diligent and practical with their money and what it was spent on. They'd grown up properly middle class, and they still have that mindset, in a lot of respects. My mom still coupons and knows to ask for a discount if a bottle of wine has a stain on the label. But I was spoiled by the way of my lifestyle, and by the expectations I developed about the world based on that lifestyle — my sister and I didn't just "get whatever we wanted," though. Sure, I didn't have to worry about buying clothes, or what would be on my plate that evening, or if the lights would suddenly go off, but I wasn't the one with money. They made it clear that we were not to worry about the basics money buys, but we were supposed to go get our own money for the shit we wanted specific to us. I mean, we're a banking family. It comes with the turf.

When we moved back to Canada, my sister and I each negotiated a five-dollar-a-week allowance in exchange for doing chores about the house, in order to have our own money. It was about this time, shortly after we arrived, that my sister and

I started drifting apart. We just didn't seem to have much in common anymore. There were other kids now. We didn't fight. We just didn't really interact anymore. I got a raise to ten dollars a week when I went to high school. I didn't have much to buy. I'm not big on consumerism in general. I got a dog, Java. Well, *we* got a dog, but she was my responsibility.

We'd had another dog, Beckie, whom we got in Barbados (initially as a guard dog, despite her being friendly with everyone), and I absolutely loved her. I was torn apart when she died. It felt like all my travel years had been cut off with a blade. I mourned her. Properly. I learned that I feel more for animals than I do for people. Something about animals is so much more conducive to love, for me, than people. Maybe it's innocence. I love kids, too — just not so much their grown forms. I feel a need to protect. I wonder if that means anything, mental health–wise ...

Java was my responsibility. And yes, one day Java, too, would die. But that was years away. There was even a decent chance I'd die first. That's the way of life. Anything can die at any time. Maybe I would even change by the time either of us died. Maybe my outlook on life would be different. Maybe my outlook on death.

Once I started trying different substances, I soon found ten dollars a week wasn't enough to cover my taste. I had to go into business for myself.

But that's not enough to justify things, is it? I don't think so now. So where did I go wrong?

It's a question my reflection asks every time the bastard catches me unaware. Why do I look like, act like, and have the track record of a goon? Someone you cross the street to escape when you have your kids with you, and fantasize about beating down when it's just you and the girl you're seeking to impress? Well, as I have to remind myself most mornings in the mirror when I wash my post-asswipe hands, I probably had something coming my way from the get-go.

As I mentioned in passing earlier, my mother had a *very* unexpected psychotic breakdown last year. I say *very* because we always expected it'd be my dad who cracked first. He's sensitive, like me: an artist on the inside who was forced to pursue an extremely stressful career to support his family's increasingly and exponentially expensifying tastes. My mom was always the solid one. The dependable Slytherin in the family — eyes on the prize, as accurate and unwavering as the Large Hadron Collider's atom beam. Then she stopped drinking her standard several goblets of vino a day over worries about high blood pressure and cholesterol. I don't think any of us had realized the recre-dicinal dimension of her drinking — it was better than the alternative, which turned out to be a fairly worrisome and heretofore undiagnosed anxiety disorder. She stopped sleeping for months on end. I don't care if you're the love child of Einstein's intellectual fortitude and Margaret Thatcher's implacable rigidity of emotion — if you don't sleep for months straight, you're going to have a mental breakdown. Guaranteed psychosis.

After a winter of battling demons inside and outside of both of us, my mother and I can have frank heart-to-hearts now about our respective mental health issues. My dad and I had battened down the hatches and kept the family together — keeping each other as sane as possible and covering for each other in keeping my mom safe. She's helped me, and I've helped her. She's been there. She's on my level. And it's coming out in leaps and bounds that we're not alone in the family at large. All sorts of blood tangents tie me to similar stories. A depressed and heavily medicated, pre–PTSD diagnosis, PTSD-case paternal grandfather, who'd signed up to kill Nazis from an RAF Spitfire at seventeen and never looked back. Mostly because he couldn't — not without staring at a wall for weeks, zonked on Valium. A maternal great-grandmother who suffered the same sort of set of symptoms as my mom. A paternal uncle of unknown everything. A family tree stretching back to the mid-1600s, full of annotations about executions, imprisonments, exiles, and all sorts of unhappy endings. A sprinkling of cousins dealing with their own issues. And then the comparatively kind, though in no way benevolent, trials and tribulations faced by the odd "normals," who were never clinically diagnosed and medicated.

And we're the one percent. Whenever I slide through a mystically beautiful valley of good, pure emotions, like empathy and gratitude, my levity is interrupted by the impossibly intrusive "What about the rest of us?" My broader family. The human race's worth of shortened finish lines and sunstroke victims — those of us facing the same issues as I am, who don't have a pillow of affordable prescriptions to fall back on, no family to trade duties with while one takes a turn for the worse, no friends for when all you need is a sensible smile on a familiar face.

* * *

Group sessions make me feel horrible about myself, but it's a good sort of sick. It's cathartic. They expose me to all sorts of people. Not all of them good, granted — some more monstrous than me — but all interesting, unique (once you get past our obvious similarities), and, largely, in more dire straits than I am. That's not to say their mental illnesses are *worse* than mine, just their situations. Actually, I would say with some degree of expertise, having passed through many and varied stages and incarnations of mental illness in my own experience, all mental illnesses are equally bad.

A psychodynamic psychotherapist once asked me over a pint at a pub what was worse, depression or mania: he'd just shared with me that he had dealt with depression in his own life, so he could understand that dimension of his patient base, but not the psychotics or manics, not in the same way. I said, falsely but with confidence, that mania was worse. In retrospect, I think I only said that because I was hypomanic at the time, on the way up: it was a closer realm of understanding than depression, which seemed a distant memory, a nice, sleepy retreat from my present psychic inferno. Really, the *worst* mental illness is whatever it is that someone is dealing with at that precise moment.

Try as we might to create or describe an objective world, we're each doing so within our individual, subjective frameworks. The gut-wrenching, akathisia-inducing, relentless nervous energy and paranoia of anxiety are just as bad as feeling critters crawling through your skin and hearing dead loved ones tell you how you've failed them while you are psychotic, which is in turn just as bad as catatonic depression and *actually* failing your *living* loved ones. To be in any one of these such extreme mental conditions, it's impossible to snap your mind around to see the world from the other side of itself.

THIRTEEN

Retrospective on 2009

I suppose by now you can assume I have a fair amount of experience with LSD, probably one of the best-known psychedelics, aside from mushrooms, of course. A lot of people ask me about how much I've done and how crazy my trips were, what they were like, etc. Story cut short, I have no idea how much I've done over the course of my life. Thousands of tabs, whatever that means in terms of the actual granular weight of LSD.

But I do know my largest single drop was in university. I was dealing, naturally, and on a drunken night, someone I only remember in this context said:

"Yo, man, if you eat a whole sheet, I'll pay for it."

The gauntlet lay on the floor, pointing at me.

—It's one-fifty a sheet.

He must have thought I was trying to pull one over on him.
"Are you serious?"

—That's a good price, man. They're a hundred micrograms each.

His expression changed a little, from guarded to inquisitive.
"No, I mean you're gonna do it?"

—Pay me first and then I will. I'll be in no shape to handle a transaction after I eat it.

He looked genuinely worried, even through the gin fog he had going, while I was sticking to my trusty Caucasian Bajans — Kahlúa, Mount Gay Rum, and milk — my own creation. Was he more worried about me than I was? I hardly knew this guy. He pulled out his wallet and handed me three fifties, and I chopped a sheet out of a page, folded it up, and put it in my mouth. I had to drink a lot of water to get that wad down, but down it went, and I went about my night.

I can't say it was the most intense experience of my life; though, by all measures, eating ten milligrams of LSD should fundamentally change a person. One thing people have noticed is that I no longer really seem to blink. My eyes self-lubricate. When I was a kid, I blinked all the time, to the point that it became a nervous tic, then I started making weird squeaking sounds, at which point I was put on mild Tourette's medication. But that's beside the point. I've noticed several of my other psychonaut friends sharing this trait of not blinking. Maybe we're just always crying.

I'm not usually a very visual person. Most of my thought is processed verbally, so I don't usually focus much on the visual aspects of most psychedelics unless they're particularly pronounced. I do, however, have 20/10 vision on a bad day. As I look out my window, I can see individual leaves on the trees a two-minute walk away. Maybe it's partly because of this that I ignore visual stimuli so much. It's too much for me. I get overwhelmed easily by sensory inputs. But every once in a while, I surrender myself to sight.

The gist of the trip was amethyst. Bronze fawns dancing on hindquarters with flutes, just like fauns with human faces gone, and cute patterned polka-dot peculiars running along their dorsal sides like pixelated prawns. Simultaneous twirling, twisting, mystic triptychs of triskelions of past, present, and beyond erupted and blended together and came blazing back and spinning faster at me than lawn mower blades gone wrong. Mowing an overgrown mind. Occam's razor shaving the Hanlon's razor stubble from my psyche. The wild spiral identity of ancient ancestry beckons heavily to me during tryptamine experiences ... especially LSD. It's even present in my beard — a spiral on either side of my throat. Its beauty takes my breath away at times. I felt connected to a neolithic proto-artist eating ergot and scrawling this strange shape in the dirt before St. Anthony's fire took them. A martyr to the cause. The earliest acid victim. Chartreuse intrudes on cobalt blues and cerise battles with cyan beneath viridian trees while lemon bees surround the scene before setting over cerulean seas.

Intense and monumental mental events collapsed into colours like a fallen Fabergé egg in a Yayoi Kusama infinity room as those blades of past, present, and future tenses receded until they ceased to make sense. In suspense, I felt I was meant to have bent myself that far — really folded that envelope, licked the stamp, and dropped it off.

Nothing to scoff at but not really that special. It was recreational. Not spiritual, or medicinal, or therapeutic. I just got really, really, really high.

Altogether, I remember it being no more powerful than taking two thousand micrograms, which I'd done before — it just lasted a bit longer, and the after-effects stretched out for about a month. To be sure, it was intense, and I took a lot from it at the time, but in the grand scheme of things, I didn't have the opportunity to integrate much of the information being downloaded into me by the massive amounts of this perennial mystery molecule. It was a typical extreme dose of LSD experience. There's no way to really categorize that, or if there were, it would be its own library, and I simply don't have the space or time to describe to the uninitiated what sorts of things go on in that mind space. I don't necessarily endorse trying it, though. This shit ain't for just anyone. Do your research. Don't make the mistakes we had to.

* * *

One of the more intense experiences of my life was much earlier than university. I was at a high-school party, where someone gave me a beer ... so I drank the beer. Duh. But as I took the last swig, I noticed something in my cup. Some paper. Some perforated paper. I pulled it out and counted twelve individual stamp-like shapes. Oh dear. I was dosed. But I was also too young to fully comprehend the scale of the dosing or what I should perhaps have done once I'd been dosed.

Yet in retrospect, I'm fairly certain that whatever was on that blotter paper was not LSD, or it was poorly manufactured LSD, or something. Because I've never had something like this happen since.

I went to the bathroom to piss. So far so good. No rainbows shooting out my dick or anything (I had no idea what to expect). I went to wash my hands and splash some water on my face, which I noticed felt lovely. I looked at myself in the mirror and felt something different from the typical strange sensation I get from looking in the mirror. I recognized that guy, but I knew he was different from me ... but which of us was in charge of this situation? I gave him a hard eye, and he gave it right back. He had beautiful eyes. Actually, all of him was beautiful. He was smiling now.

—Can I look at your eyes closer?

Sure, he seemed to respond.

I leaned in and studied his fluctuating pupil size, then panned outward to the rest of the eye. He had a close, short ring of browns and blacks and oranges that bunched below a thin ring of gold and yellow before blooming into a green canopy through the rest of his iris. It looked like a forest bent around a ring. I wondered if he was having a similar experience.

—Can I come in?

Sure, he seemed to welcome.   ·

The transition from narcissistic bathroom-mirror studying to being a seed dropped from one of those trees in the forest was seamless. The drug gods played their cards well.

I germinated, my roots sank into the mycelial black hole network of my pupils, then I reached for the light. Seasons cycled through the rings that ran around my centre. I added them annually to my vegetal soul vessel, growing up and out. I became a mother tree. I distributed nutrients to my fellow eyes. I watched the wildlife seemingly rush by compared to what felt like my centuries of experience. The time scale of the creatures seemed glancingly brief. I was glad to be a tree. I became an entity beyond the scope of your average tree. I had the right genes, and I landed in the right place, and I wasn't chewed up by bugs

or critters in my adolescence. I was a landmark. I became a
sacred place for the creatures that came into my forest, chasing
out the bears and wolves. They burned my fallen branches in
some form of ritual. I have no idea how long I spent as a tree,
but it was a transformative experience. Walking through forests
has changed in its qualities since this trip.

 The next stage of the experience, though, was a bit more
jarring:

acid-based drain wash

```
check yourself in the mirror,
man: asking what happened to that paper
covered in shit. here one minute, then
   gone
and the cartoons are on, too. flickering
through a slit in this door to the other
room is some sort of strobe light, like
   inside
clubs with no bathrooms inside
where you have to pack a pocket mirror
for perspective on your pupils. other
from that you're alone, just thoughts
   and paper
smashing together, old flint flickering
finally: finely folded fire. gone
like, dissolved on your tongue, gone
like that person you always were, inside
someone else's self: faded, flickering
to a point. disappeared by the mirror.
vomit in a full sink of burnt paper
and try to turn the knob for the other
guy outside the door, other-
wise he might be, well, nothing worse
   than gone
```

to get help. but, you still need the paper
only you can't find it, though it's
   inside
for sure. except, don't look through the
   mirror
or else you'll never stop that
   flickering
reflected in flickering
reflexes kicking in as another
version of you climbs out of the mirror
and no matter how hard you look, it's
   gone
because you need to try searching inside
not just on your pretty picture paper.
forget about the paper
and follow the source of the flickering
away from the toilet you're stuck inside
since, sooner or later, you know other
people need to use it, and need you gone
so they can spend some time in their
   mirror.
give up on the paper and the other
flickering pictures that all end up gone
the moment you move inside the mirror.

   I found myself somewhere safe, and I rode it out clutching
a pillow, giggle-crying and talking to anything I thought could
hear me.

FOURTEEN

Retrospective on 2002

I remember the first time I got high very, very clearly. High on weed, I mean ... nothing crazy. Not just yet. I was about twelve, and I brought some home from school that I'd traded for a dick-shaped steel lighter I found in French class. I gathered my two buddies who lived on the street and were roughly in my age bracket, and we all convinced our parents to let us have a sleepover. One of the guys was bringing some amazing Polish chocolate from his parents' deli. We needed entertainment, though, to boost this gnarly looking green and orange mess of leaves, or so we'd heard. I'd been given the perfect idea of what to get high to for the first time by the guy who gave me the schwag:

"I wish I'd done Dark Side of Oz my first time."

This guy was a stoner to the core: long hair, tie-dyed socks in pleather sandals, sarcastic while stupid; he must know his shit. His fuckin' name was Gutter, for chrissakes.

He pulled the stuff out of his pocket, picked a bit of lint out, and passed it to me.

—Do you have a bag?

"Does it look like I have a bag?"

We waited until the parents of the kid whose house we were staying at fell asleep, then we migrated from the basement to the kitchen and back, set up with all the Doritos and Sour Patch Kids we could see needing. Then we set up the experience. There's a precise timing when you have to start playing Pink Floyd's *Dark Side of the Moon* in synchronicity with *The Wizard of Oz* to get it to match up, but when you get it ... well ... it's trippy.

I'm sorry if you aren't familiar with Dark Side of Oz. Wait, no, I'm not. It's iconic. Put down the book for a moment and look it up. Smoking a bowl first won't hurt ...

So we opened the basement window and felt the keen winds of January as we huddled around it. We smoked the pot out of an apple, like the dealer told me, since I wasn't sure if I'd like it and I didn't want to invest in a pipe. It tasted like warlock ass ... probably mouldy, in retrospect, but we managed to cough most of it out the window ... we were probably fine. It couldn't smell that much. The other two sank into their spots, and I followed suit after pressing the appropriate buttons and dimming the lights.

The screaming at the beginning of the album was mixing with the tornado in a really disconcerting way — I mean, *really* disconcerting. I felt broken. The walls were closing in. This was gonna be forever, wasn't it? I was clutching my face with no memory of moving my arms. The screaming intensified and grew and coalesced into a monument of terror, then it broke. Next comes that lovely, floaty, easy breezy Zen garden of sound one minute and ten seconds into "Speak to Me/Breathe," the first song off *Dark Side of the Moon.*

I was home. Not physically. Mentally, spiritually, emotionally. How had I lived without this? How could I go on living without this? This was sublime. I finally understood half of Sublime's songs. My mind ran like a rabbit all throughout "Breathe" just like they were telling it to — what groovy lyrics Floyd had.

We ate all our munchies in the first half hour or so, Polish chocolate decorated with winged hussars beating back our encroaching hunger. I got up off an ottoman, and we went upstairs and ran into the kid's older sister. I had a crush on her. That was awkward. But hunger prevailed! We decided to make instant oatmeal. We debated which was better: apple cinnamon or maple and brown sugar. We got it ready.

"Guys, you can't microwave spoons."

—Ohhhh. Riiiight.

"Are you guys OK?"

—Yeaaah.

"Uh huh."

"Toootally."

I look at both of my buddies' bloodshot eyeballs and assumed I was sporting the same look.

"OK. Have fun … Stay safe."

Cool sister.

I invested in a shitty little screw-together metal pipe a few days later. The same one everyone smokes through their first time.

FIFTEEN
January 2008

Midnight in the garden between good and evil.

Tonight we trip! Six of us assemble: Goof, Munchkin, Cozy the Dwarf, Weasel, Village Idiot, and me ... whatever my name would be. We've found ourselves congregated in a dorm room in midwinter with a dangerous combination of no purpose, nothing to do, and too many substances. It quickly became apparent they shared my overwhelming urge to have a group trip of some consequence.

Yay! Group trips!

For exposition: Each person you add to a trip party varies its result in unpredictable ways. While several closely aligned minds (like, for example, a cult ... say, the Manson Family) co-experiencing meaning will often result in truly incredible outcomes, grouping six random teenagers based solely on their gender, geographical proximity, and willingness to consume just about whatever they can may have unusual endings.

The parameters of the evening are set. It will all be natural. We will follow in the footsteps of our shamanic fathers as we consume a botanical display's worth of solely psychotropic plants. The goal, should we find ourselves capable of reaching it, is to consume more substances than we have fingers to count them with. We've done our research. We have the right stuff, and in the right doses. We have homemade temple ball hash laced with opium (following in the footsteps of our hippie forebears), several varietals of magic mushrooms to give us a nice rounded out psilocybe experience, San Pedro (mescaline) tea, homemade ayahuasca of Syrian rue and *Mimosa hostilis* root bark, Hawaiian baby woodrose seeds (full of LSA, a close analogue of LSD), home-rolled cigars of *Nicotiana rustica* leaf (much stronger than traditional cultivars of tobacco), a carefully selected strain from a reputable supplier of kratom, raw salvia leaves for chewing purposes, and hobo-wine.

Yeah. Hobo-wine. Also known as toilet-wine, or afternoon-delight. We made it by opening a juice bottle, adding a bunch of sugar and a crumb of stale bread or some baker's yeast, then capping the bottle using a condom with a hole poked through. The hole was to let carbon dioxide from the fermentation process out, while keeping out bacteria and contaminants. We're actually pretty good at it.

We also each fill up a Thermos of thick, syrupy Ethiopian coffee to keep us warm in the negative twenty-odd Celsius cold and to spark us up should something else drag us down.

Let's start this in earnest. I slam all the classic tryptamines within about half an hour of each other, knowing that their tolerance windows overlap. I'm gobbling unmeasured handfuls of mushrooms, crushing fifteen Hawaiian baby woodrose seeds in my teeth, and steeling myself against the godawful tastes. I'm gulping down these handfuls of madness with alternating brews of ayahuasca and San Pedro tea, stopping very glancingly to cleanse my palate with hobo-wine. I wonder, *What would Jesus do?* and decide emphatically he'd do exactly what I'm doing: getting close to God.

With the core components of the trip now unsettlingly crammed into my stomach, I've pretty much removed myself psychically from the crowd. I make myself some kratom before the contents of my guts can come to life and hurl me into the unknown. As the medicines begin seeping into my system, I coax them deeper with breaths of wild-tobacco cigars, alternating with the hookah full of hash mixed with opium. I drift deeper into this swishing, listless, aimless, drifting, cosmic laziness of psychoplasmic blahness for a while.

"Let's go outside!"

—No.

"Yeah, let's go to the arboretum!"

Have they not been taking the same drugs I have? It's fucking freezing outside. You don't need mescaline to show you the Mandelbrot flakes forming on the windowpanes.

—Cold. No. Cold. Stay.

"Yeah. Let's go to the Zen garden."

My arguments aren't as well put-together as theirs are, so the group decides to go for a stroll. I use the opportunity to take my tenth entheogen for the walk, though, scooping up a bundle of *Salvia divinorum* leaves and stuffing them in my gums on the way out the door. I hold my Ethiopian coffee near. It's very cold out.

The coinciding, colliding varieties of psychedelia surround me in a cyclone of patterns and what looks like paints and gemstones and stained-glass motifs, mosaics of Aztec pictograms, Dalian wax melting from every surface, the calculus of zeroes and infinities stretched out on polygonal playing matrices, spirals of unsung colours coming off of every fucking thing. This is art. This is all art. This moment, the whole of it, is art. So is this moment. So is every moment. Life is art. Art is life. Is that what my life is? Art? Is that why I'm an artist? The information encoded in the realities presented to me is scrambling my usual cranial static. This is a level beyond the scope of the ordinary day tripper. I've passed into the realms of 8A and B geometry, simultaneously.

Geometry of the 8A variety is more commonly associated with a drug like LSD; 8B with mushrooms. There are similarities in the nature of the effects to the casual observer, but the experience is extremely variable, and the two forms of geometry can be quite dissonant.

I think of it this way: 8A lays out an infinite array of data points presented to your third eye by digitized visual representations of stimuli with semantic connecting nodes; when your mind lands on something, you spread out to everything that original point is related to. You spiderweb your experience. It's very "do your own thing."

The 8B kind definitely seems to have more of an agenda. At this point, the drug is trying to tell you something, and you'd better listen. Truth is encoded in every layer of the notepad of your life you flip through, thumbing through the papercuts, too. No matter where you turn, the message of the trip persists: you *will* learn from this.

"Dudes, don't step on the sand! It'll disturb the trees!"

Cozy the Dwarf is standing on a squat Japanese-inspired, Shinto-style statue in the middle of the Zen garden. A clear path of footprints leads through the snow to the base of the statue. I guess he must be fairly well past gone, too. Looking around I sum up the expeditionary party: Cozy is standing guard against the spirits; Goof still hasn't made it into the garden, confounded by the little bridge over a frozen koi pond; Munchkin is playing with unscooped dog poop; Weasel is walking in circles around the garden, making sure to step only in his own footprints; and Village Idiot is just staring perplexed back at me, half his fist shoved in his mouth and dripping saliva. We are the leaders of tomorrow.

The trees sway, whether due to the weather or the chemicals, whatever, and the snow looks like kodama blessing our outing. This is a good night.

But everything ends. On the way out of the Zen garden, crossing that confounding little bridge that had stymied Goof, I step off the edge and break through the ice and into the water, up to the hip in nasty-ass pond water in the middle of January. Within minutes my pants are made of small plates of icicles, and I can feel the cold everywhere. Everywhere. *Everywhere.* I'm dying. This is what dying feels like. Everyone says it feels cold. Who's "everyone"? How many people are dying then talking about how cold it was? Ludicrous. Is this what you think about as you die? The same inane shit you think about while you live? That can't be right. I can't be dying. I have to be more poetic when I die.

—Am I dying?

"Man. I dunno. I'm fucked. Have some hobo-wine. Warm up."

Right! My Ethiopian coffee! Warmth! I chug half the coffee, then rub the other half over my freezing legs. The temporary heat is scalding, but the ensuing warmth is delightful. The long-term point is non-existent. I'm immediately cold again ... just covered in coffee grounds. I am, though, wired. The moon has tracers. So does every single star. Swaying my head gently has the effect of staring at a trillion spinning sparkler sticks.

Then suddenly, I gotta get back. I wanna go to bed. I need to be in bed. I wanna be safe.

This is a tall order, as we're about a twenty-minute walk from our dorm and, as I think is clear by now, not at our best. Something like three or four hours later, nearing frostbite on my toes, we breach the door of our dorm. We pile into the elevator and press floor four, and the door closes.

"Is it warm in here?"

"Yeah, man. It's fuckin' hot."

I can't tell who just spoke. I don't care. I can feel it rising. It's in my toe tips, coming from the freezing and spreading throughout my lower body, latching onto my tailbone and launching itself up my Kundalini nerve of awareness before blasting me with the obvious. The heat is on. I strip my January-appropriate garments in earnest. Psychedelia can be very temperature dependent, and I find that rapidly jacking the thermostat can really send a trip into hyperspace. Especially a bad trip.

I don't know who I am. I'll never know, and I don't think I want to know. I'm scared that I'm inherently a bad person, or that the sum of my actions makes me a bad person, and I'm scared to look closely from either a subjective or objective lens. I've done so, so many bad things, but I've done good things, too, right? And most of my thoughts are good thoughts, most of the time, but that doesn't go far in the court of public opinion. This might be the path to a *true* name, my magic name, but that might just be a curse.

Follow your nightmares. They mean more than your dreams.

We hit the fourth floor and spill out, six eighteen-year-old boys, averaging well over two hundred pounds apiece, with a mini-monsoon from sweat forming behind us. We pass Mary, our residence assistant, an older, responsible student who's stayed in the dorms to keep us youngsters out of trouble.

"Hey guys, how are you? You look rough."

More than a few of the substances we've consumed cause nausea, especially when mixed in unconventional ways with each other. Brushing through her, I chuck myself through a luckily selected door and extrude my guts across the bathroom tiles. I am not subtle. This sounds like Yoko on a megaphone. Mary comes inside.

"Are you all right?"

Ahahahahahahaha. What the fuck? Is that a question? Her look of concern is folding into a loop. Her face, seemingly made of Play-Doh, is salsa dancing with my delirium and pre-existing crush on her.

You know how when a wheel or propellor gets going really, really fast, there comes a point where it almost looks like it's going slowly in reverse? This starts happening to the floor of diagonally checkered black and white tiles, with a large central, amoeba-looking globule of vomit as a geographical focal point. The puke is spinning and spinning, and suddenly spinning blurrily backwards in a most disconcerting way. Then something changes, and the puke begins speeding up to the point that it becomes even blurrier, reduces speed again, and reverses direction. How am I moving this fast? Am I going in one direction or spinning in opposite directions concurrently? Is that possible? That's stupid. Anything's possible. You just have to believe anything's possible. Start marching in the direction you believe the possibility lies, and put in the work, right? That's how people do things? That's how we put people on the moon. They said it was impossible. That's how we make vaccines. You assume it's possible, then you get to work. Vaccines. They're for sick people. No, they're to stop you from getting sick. I haven't been vaccinated for anything in a while. Am I sick right now?

—Flu.

"Oh, jeez."

She backs off, and my sweating, dilated pupils, and erratic behaviour are now explainable to some degree. The guys get me into my room, and I go under a blanket for the next six or so hours, with no discernible memory of what has happened during these six or so hours once I exit this soft, bland, beige comforter as my mind starts clearing up. We all generally emerge from our safe places at around the same time, then go for breakfast. None of us are particularly talkative. All any of us has the stomach for is two-litre cartons of whole milk ... so we sit in the common area, chugging fatty milk and ruminating gently in hushed tones over the pros and cons of the night.

"Yeah, I'm not doing that again."

"Same."

"Me too, man."

"I never want to do drugs again."

"That was pretty cool."

Goof is, well, a fucking imbecile.

—Fuck no.

I'm freaked. Freaky freaked. There were points in the trip where I forgot I was on drugs, which is just about one of the worst directions your brain can take while on fuckloads of drugs. I thought I was going, going, gone. There are bad trips and terror trips. A lot of people think they've had a horrible experience on psychedelics when really it was just a difficult chapter of the trip; maybe they were confronted by a particularly ugly truth about themselves, and they had difficulty integrating that to their world view. Maybe it could've been averted with a trip-sitter, or a bit more research, or an openness to the challenges that psychedelics can pose to the ego. That's just part of the game. But sometimes you have a far, far worse experience. Time broke down completely. I did, too, trapped in a cuckoo clock with twisted and jagged gears all around me.

I contact a few middlemen I know and lay out the terms: I just want my drugs gone and at least some of my money back. I clear out of everything. All my weed, mushrooms, acid, and strange one-offs. I barely make back my investment, but I'm happy to just not have that sort of heat on me — both the legal aspect and the fact that I have a very hard time not doing drugs once they're in my possession. So I'm cleaned out. I'm gonna focus on school. I'm gonna take some philosophy courses, too, at some point. I need to formally study weird thoughts rather than just jumping headfirst into another cocktail of cerebral composting.

SIXTEEN

Retrospective on 2015

After a period of convalescence following my legal troubles, I decided to try my hand at a legal career route. At the suggestion of a neighbour of my parents, who was the president of a major publishing firm and took note of my keen interest in reading and writing, I enrolled in a publishing course in 2013. He took me out for pints to extol the virtues of publishing.

"It can be a launch pad to politics, or journalism, or your own writing. And I gotta tell you, you're a fine young man. You've got a bright future. It's an industry predominantly populated by young women. And some of them are gorgeous. You could have the pick of the litter, buddy."

Seedy. I see this guy driving his kids to the cottage every weekend, but these sorts of fellas are in every industry.

Editing did seem like a job right up my alley, though. What could be better than reading about new things every day? Learning from a wide array of topics and perspectives is built into the job description. I followed the program with an internship at a small publisher based out of Toronto. I loved it.

A tiny little building space stacked with books, soon-to-be books, and words incongruously welded together into intellectually immobile objects the authors of which called "books" (but that never would be). These already cramped quarters were divided into three walk-in closet–type mini-offices where lived the editor, publicist, and miscellaneously untitled dude who did a bit of everything; these were all connected by a larger forum, in which I sat directly across from the Publisher.

Hello, boss.

With no opportunity to slack off (under the keen gaze of the Publisher), I put in my true amount of potential. I tried. I cared to try. I started off doing proofreading: checking the final drafts for typos, making sure the page numbers added up, etc. I quickly proved capable of more challenging tasks, and soon I was editing properly.

A copy of a manuscript hit my desk in the morning. It was due at the printer two days prior. My only job was to give it a final look-over and approve it on the way out the door. I got to work in earnest, paying close attention to every detail — marking out the errors as I saw them come up. There seemed to be a lot of errors, and pretty early on in the book. I started skimming. Typo, tense shift, unclear who's speaking in the dialogue ... then started the big issues. "Wasn't that character called something else earlier in the book? Isn't this scene out of character for the protagonist? Uhh ... I thought that character was dead." I skipped lunch to keep reading and brought up to the Publisher a list of errors too long to be fixed with typography. So many continuity errors, stylistic incongruities, people showing up out of nowhere and going nowhere. How this escaped the multiple layers of editing to get to this point was beyond comprehension to either of us.

"We have to fix this. Before it goes to the printers. This is garbage as is."

—What should we do? Can you get in contact with the author?

"They're on vacation in the Bahamas. They thought this was done. We're going to have to do something about this."

—What's "something"?

Something turned out to be a full-body massaging of the literary knots back into the fabric of the greater storyline. We worked late that night. I got an acknowledgement in the novel, which was genuinely a good book, and I was so proud.

Getting into the grit of the storyline, analyzing the characters for consistency, revising stylistic missteps on the part of the author. I was working side by side with the publisher and respected for my input as a valuable member of the team: my initial internship was extended another three months. I could definitely see myself enjoying this career.

This also happened to be a period over which I'd been experimenting with psychedelics in a way new to me. I was microdosing. I wasn't doing any other drugs, just LSD or psilocybe mushrooms. Well, MDMA once or twice. Oh, and weed. Always weed. I would eat between 0.3 and 0.6 grams of mushrooms, depending on the species, or fifteen to twenty-five micrograms of LSD every four to seven days. Sometimes I would mix them, finding they interacted in an interesting way ... the acid stretches out the mushrooms and the mushrooms mellow out the acid. I'd seen some papers and heard stories, mostly anecdotal — but that's all you usually get so far for psychedelics (except for the golden age before they were illegalized, when they were touted in thousands of papers as breakthrough medications for all sorts of physical and psychiatric issues) — that microdosing in this fashion could help to improve creativity, mood, stability, focus ... all that good shit. I wasn't exactly surprised when I found the effects to be pretty much as described.

Having done massive doses of these same chemicals where phenomenal, seemingly divine, always life-changing experiences followed, I could tell that smaller doses could potentially have beneficial properties. I was in an elevated state ... not quite hypomanic per se, but borrowing all the best parts of it. I was prolific and creative, exercising, focusing on my diet, more in touch with my emotions, patient with people, insightful and energetic, but able to meditate myself to sleep. I was better. I was what I wanted to be. This was like finding weed all over again. The one thing I'll say, call it a tip, is to take a lower dose of psychedelic and then titrate your experience with cannabis, which mixes excellently with classic tryptamines in safe conditions. I'm not sure whether it was the microdosing, the internship, or both simultaneously giving me stability, but this period of five months was one of the best of my life to date.

Then the internship ended.

Unfortunately, with print publishing not exactly having its heyday of late, there was no permanent position waiting for me on the back end of the internship, no matter how hard I worked to be impressive. I applied to any place I could in the publishing industry, but positions were scant and often filled through nepotism or networkers before the call for resumés even went out. I got one interview for the hundred or so applications I made over a few months.

"It says on your resumé that you're proficient in Photoshop and InDesign? Do you have those programs already down-loaded on your laptop?"

—Yes, I do. Unfortunately, though, they're pirated versions, which have served my purposes just fine so far, but I'm not sure if you'd need me to download the official versions?

Fairly innocuous comment, I thought.

"Did you just admit, in an interview, for a publisher, to stealing intellectual information? Are you serious? Do you really think you'll get this job now? Is there any more point to this interview?"

We obviously have very different ethical foundations.

—Well, those programs cost more than my entire publishing course, and you're offering minimum wage even if I got the job. And I don't think Adobe really misses a few thousand dollars the same desperate way you miss a five-dollar pirated ebook. Would you cover the cost of my getting the programs, or does a few thousand bucks for a computer program seem a bit steep to you, too, and you'd just rather I cover it? Is the work produced for you to be strictly financed by your employees?

I didn't get the job. I stopped sending out applications. Instead I turned my attention to my own writing.

I've always written poetry and stories, and it's been a dream to just be able to write for the rest of my life, but I was never really plugged into the writing world the way you need to be to get one of those gigs. I'd studied biology and philosophy, not literature or English. And, minor point, I didn't read much "literature." Oh sure, I read a lot of books as a kid, but not many of the classics, and practically zero contemporary Canadian literature (a must in order to schmooze your way through the CanLit community).

I had a lot of interests as a kid — history, geography, politics ... the physical sciences and math, astronomy, philosophy — but they'd faded over the course of my university and publishing years. Maybe it's because those were precisely the topics I'd studied and worked on in the years since first being enamoured by them. The magic and mystery had burned itself out. I felt robbed. And for what? I was pissed. I wanted to get back at academia. I wanted to throw up both my middle fingers on a page and nail it to the doors of the institutes of the intelligentsia. I wanted to show up the stuck-up fucks who'd shut me down.

And poetry? I hate most poetry that I've read. Just awful. So I set about trying to do better. My internship had exposed me to a whirlwind of artfully constructed prose and passable poetry, and I was swept up with ideas and techniques completely foreign to me. I wanted to use that as a springboard for my own writing career. I wrote a series of poems and spoken word pieces, and I put out a homemade chapbook in the winter of 2014. A few friends bought pity copies, and the rest went on my shelf. I forgot about writing and editing for a few months as another wave of depression rippled across me.

* * *

I watch myself a lot. I mean, in the mirror — and videos, yeah, yeah, videos. And like, I listen to my own music. Is that vain? No. No, I don't think so. Also, I read my written shit: over and over and over and — I try to perfect it, that's all. That's what I'm trying to do. I want to make it perfect! You see, I'm just trying to relate to reality. I'm coming at things sideways all the time. I want a perpendicular inversion. I want belonging. And I want belonging to want me. I study myself like a subject I could connect with because the teacher was cool. I seek out patterns, like how many steps ahead of the rest equates to acing the next big test, or how much time at a desk makes me a teacher's pet? I'd grow myself a fucking apple orchard if I thought my approval could be bought with sweet taste and no texture; I'd stew a sea of cider when they turned out sour — but I'm not a generous drunk. When I spin my perspective like a lucky penny flipped to make a quick, split-second, permanent decision, I just criticize myself creatively.

So it's back to beating myself into being the Me in some abstract, paranoid-paralysis, parallax-refracted, machine-minded mask of sanity. But, you know, it's all for the love of poetry: my rosary bead on a never-ending rotary phone trying repeatedly to place a call to the sanatorium orderly. A deformity. A malady my ancestry and aggressive assault of tactical psychonautic artillery has encoded me with. And I live with it because I love my masochistic mystic side: it mystifies me with its solipsist, sadistic evil eye.

Now, I'm pretty notorious for never going out without a notebook and a back-up pen in my pocket. I sit in stereotypical settings, like Starbucks or subway seats, and beat out little, chicken-scratch scribbles on sheets of sterile sketch paper (because I like the thickness and the way it soaks up calligraphy ink). People often ask me about the sorts of stuff I write: Is it fiction? A play script? Is it a song? Is it funny or sad? Have you been doing this long? Just a journal for you? Or is it meant to be read? I hope it's not poetry ... 'cause, you know, everything you can think has been said and poetry's dead.

You may hear a poem, but do you feel it?

You might let this language leak with listless laziness along your cerebellum's symbolic hot spots, seeking solely sexual stimuli in the sound of it, but do you feel the contours of a letter? Does it tickle your timid, typically off-limits, nether regions like a feather painting pleasure-purpose private parts and neural paths with pain-inducing chili peppers? Get you whether it's in leather or wearing silk and making soothing, moving, pre-human, pelvic-grooving gestures? Let the phonetics stick themselves, for better or worse, within your sacred centre and vibrate there forever like subatomic strings charged by the power of "In the beginning was the Word"?

I usually lose them somewhere soon after the second sentence — but that's the sickness involved in this psychotically obsessive, solitary second sentence:

I MUST NOT FAIL! I MUST NOT FAIL! I MUST NOT FAIL! I MUST NOT FAIL! I MUST NOT FAIL! I —

SEVENTEEN

Retrospective on Spring 2014

One of my friends ended up giving his copy of my chapbook to his father, a prominent psychiatrist, because of the poetry's central focus on mental health issues. His father put it on his shelf in his office, which was fortunate for my career as he just so happened to be the doctor of another writer of poetry: an older, more experienced writer. A writer with a published book. A real writer. My friend's father asked if he could give the chapbook and my contact information to the writer, who we'll just call the Godfather for this story's purposes. I agreed whole-heartedly, excited at the prospect of possibly meeting someone who might be able to guide my outsider artist aesthetic toward something a bit more marketable. He was a poet, which is the kind of writing I'd been focusing more on of late, and I was curious to see what an established, informed, and, most of all, classically trained writer would say about my work.

It was about a month until I heard from my friend's father that the Godfather had actually seen enough merit in my material to want to meet up. For some reason, my friend's father, the psychiatrist treating the Godfather, gave me the Godfather's contact information and told me to reach out to him. Hadn't I already given him my contact information? Is this just writer etiquette or something? The newbie has to be the one who reaches out?

No. It was just him.

I bought a bottle of wine and brought my usual pipe and Baggie of pot (just in case he was cool) to meet him and his partner, another emerging writer in the Toronto scene. They were really nice. He was definitely, well, kooky, but they both seemed well intentioned. He opened up that he was being treated for bipolar disorder and had recently been discharged from hospital after ten years of being in the wards. We bonded on a mental health level. After a slice of pie, the Godfather suggested the two of us go for a stroll to discuss my writing.

"Hey, man, do you smoke weed, man?"

—Oh, dude, I'm so happy you asked that. I've been aching to smoke a bowl.

"Here, man, let's use mine. I have a pipe. It's the only one I use."

—Nice. Thanks, man. After I brought the bottle of wine and we didn't open it, I didn't really know what was going on.

I'd brought the unopened wine with us because, well, what's the point in leaving it?

—Do you want any wine?

"I don't really drink, man. Want some coke? Just don't tell my girlfriend. I love her so much, man, but she doesn't understand this sort of thing. I have to protect her."

Fuckin' right.

I woke up the next day on their couch with the taste of red wine vomit in my mouth and the stuffed, stinging sinuses that follow a night of snorting heavily cut blow. Quite the introduction to the Canadian literary community. This was going to be a fun summer.

EIGHTEEN
Summer 2014

This is not a conventional education in poetics. About five days a week, I meet up with the Godfather for a sort of writing camp. I'm treating this like a full-time job, and it's taking its toll.

I'm tired as fuck. This is more intense than any work-position I've had. Way more intense than publishing school, or even university — not in the drug sense, either — just the sheer volume of work I'm putting out, the lack of sleep, the feeling of encroaching mania. I'm losing weight, and sometimes it feels like I'm losing my mind. Maybe this is just how the Godfather teaches. "Embrace the insanity."

The Godfather said that he'd enjoyed the passion, language, and subject matter of my chapbook but pointed out that, having essentially a layman's insights on the mechanics of writing a poem, I could certainly benefit from learning something a bit more familiar to readers. I'm going to learn *forms*.

The Godfather's preferred method of instruction is to bring a Baggie of coke to the bar/park/house we end up at, name an obscure form of poetry, share a bump, then tell me to look it up and write one in an hour; then we have another bump and go over the poem, him pointing out the merits and pitfalls, my mind too abuzz to process any of the few lessons I'm learning. Cocaine is definitely an integral part of this whole process. Luckily, he's buying.

The Godfather has a sort of fetishization of death and early blowouts in an artist's prime, like Rimbaud or Nelligan, that I identify strongly with. I never expected to make it past eighteen. I've felt like I'm on borrowed time since then. One thing we differ on, though, is his glorification of mania. He's addicted to it. I'm just dealing with it. I don't want to glory in it.

This is a period of frenzied writing for me. Largely drug-fueled, as is clear by now, but I must say, it's producing some of my favourite poems so far. Villanelles, pantoums, ghazals, sestinas, glosas: these forms fascinate me. I find that the censorship of movement forces creativity in ways a blank canvas simply can't. My creativity is blossoming in the confines of my mentor's incessant form of formal poetics, forcing forms on me until I am formed in his fashion.

* * *

Then I found my own voice and burst out. I wasn't just a poet, I was a writer, of everything ... I wrote art ... whatever the fuck that meant.

One night we were writing in a park, sharing bumps, me occasionally spouting a spoken word poem I'd been writing shortly before this education in formal poetics began. The Godfather didn't approve of that type of poetry, being obsessed as he was with the concept of forms and the immortality of the printed word. He was old school like that. A bit on the conservative side, for an artist; he reminded me of a devoutly Catholic, conspiracy-adhering mob boss. Not necessarily a contradiction in terms ... just, he set an unusual precedent. Dude was a walking paradox, in a lot of ways. Fiendishly brilliant in how he could weave words into intricate lace patterns, but totally incapable of finding his way home or generally interacting with the world at large.

He seemed to take umbrage with the neurotypical. He wanted a revolution of the mad. I don't think he had any plans for what would happen after madness ruled.

There was nothing particularly untoward about the look of the guy, except he never wore socks ... even, like, in black leather shoes. I thought that was odd. Well, it stands out in my memory. He had a dense mop of thick, curly black hair sitting on top of his skull, with a week-long shadow stretched across his chin and around his nose. A little overweight, but I'll put that down to the meds. He was keen to show me pictures of when he'd been in his twenties. He was a damn good-looking guy.

* * *

Seemingly out of nowhere, the Godfather turns to me with an unspecified, vague sort of terror in his face:

"Dude, I can't find the coke."

—Oh shit.

"Did you take my coke?"

Ah fuck. The last thing I need is to be labelled a coke thief. I didn't take the coke. Though, that would've been a good idea. But definitely not from my one human link to what I like to imagine might one day possibly be a career in writing … like, ideally.

—No, man, I swear. I'll buy another bag if you want. I just won't be able to get it tonight.

"No, it's OK, man. I didn't actually believe you took it."

That's a lie. Coke stimulates your baser instincts. Once the idea gets in your head, it's very hard to get out. But he must not believe, just be reserving suspicion. If he actually believed I'd stolen it, there would be hell to pay. Don't fuck with an addict's drugs. I have to somehow prove that I'm as dispirited as he is, it being his coke.

"Let's spread out and look."

I look out over the field. There are two baseball diamonds and a dog park, and we've been walking around the whole time. What else can I do? I need a foothold in the writing world.

—OK.

We look for about three hours in silence, except for when I ask the dog walkers near the baseball diamond if, by chance, they've seen a little bag full of white powder. No? Worth a shot. I check the bleachers, at the Godfather's request, even though we haven't even sat on them; he thinks maybe someone else has taken it, then they might have lost it. I search to mollify him. I wave the flashlight on my phone over the grass like a mine-sweeper until the battery dies. We don't find anything, and we both go home pissed off and unsatisfied.

* * *

Another perk of having a writing "mentor" is the access it grants you. I was finally meeting writers I'd heard about. I was going to all sorts of launches and readings and brunches and learning that this is a very "I'll scratch your back" industry. Good thing I have long nails. Still, even to me, it seems desperate. I can see, however, that there are crossover skills from selling drugs that might work well in entertainment. Like self-promotion.

One thing I noticed early on — and in conferring with the Godfather my suspicions crystallized — many of these other writers have turned mental illness into a commodity. Being bipolar is a hot topic. Depression gets deals done. Mania is almost deified. And if you've been psychotic, why, that's just as good as being granted artistic and philosophical insights the likes of which the great unwashed could never dream.

Writers crowd around the new kid, cowing me to make their first impressions:

"To me, depression feels like, y'know, an overwhelming sadness. It's like, y'know, I don't even wanna do things. That's when I write."

Convincing. You obviously know what you're talking about.

"Oh my God, I have PTSD. Isn't that fucked up?"

That's how you introduce it? And, if you do, how does that make you unique?

"Psychosis is like … so many colours and shit."

Oh yeah? Colours? As in pouring out all the *orange* juice in the house because you suddenly believe it's been spiked with sodium pentothal by the government, to incapacitate you so they can take you in for Mengele-type experiments? Colours like believing only the *red* Christmas-cookie tins make the right frequency of vibration when they fall from their place leaned up against all the doors to alert you to any intruders in the house? Colours like *green* are what these people are. They just wanna be seen on the scene. Who cares how insincere they've been?

"My anxiety feels like butterflies in my stomach. I try to think of it as my 'cute' superpower, since it makes me work harder."

FUCK YOU! My anxiety feels like stomach acid boring holes in my belly because I haven't eaten in three days and my throat is stinging from the bile I've been vomiting. I'm shivering like Jack Dawson chillin' on a door in the North Atlantic, and I'm snapping at all of my closest allies because I'm too afraid to snap at anyone else but OH MY FUCKING GOD I HAVE TO FUCKING SNAP SOMEHOW!

Being unstable is edgy. This is all the more pertinent to me given the Godfather's book, fresh off the presses, is a series of poems all about mental health and the struggles inherent in living with bipolar disorder. I see other writers flock to him, obsequious in deference to a mental disorder on "another level" from the one they experience (or claim to, for career purposes).

"Wow. What you've been through. I can't imagine. I mean, I've been anxious and depressed before, but, like, being bipolar seems *so* much more fucked up. Do you think you *need* to have mental health issues to write poetry? Or, like, y'know, to write *good* poetry?"

Or "Have you ever noticed how many poets have mental disorders? It's like a prerequisite for our job."

Or "At least it's not schizophrenia, though. Right?"

The thing you don't notice for a little while is that, as cool as it might be to *have* an issue, it's supremely uncool to *display* an issue. It's a similar story with drugs. So many artists speak ad nauseam of their favourite drugs and trips — you know, that one time they tried MDMA, or they ate a tab of LSD, or they smoked a cannabis cigarette and "Just lost it, y'know?" Then they defer the opportunity to have a taste when I offer them some. "I don't need designer drugs. I've got a designer personality." Psychological atypicality, or the appearance thereof, is just another commodity, I guess. Everyone wants to seem special, noteworthy, there. Everyone wants to be seen at the pool party. It's a ticket to *the strange* for the connoisseur of the cliché. No one wants to come in the deep end with us, though. That's a lesson that, once learned, I very much did not dive in line with.

The Godfather invited me to a fancy, glitterati event, a publisher's fall book line launch and readings by all the authors. It was all very networking appropriate. Naturally, I sabotaged myself. Heading out from the Godfather's house, I had my requisite while-with-the-Godfather cocaine, then proceeded to down an unmeasured handful of mushrooms on the subway. By the time we arrived at the party, I had a good sweat on. These mushrooms were very — how do I describe this — gooey. Everything was sticky. The air was heavy and humid. I felt my bowels reflecting my gooey vibes.

The readings were abysmal. At least, that was my assessment while tripping balls and keeping a tight grip on my sphincter. I had to find the bathroom.

—Godfather, where do people shit?

"I know, man. All the books are absolute shit. None of them are in the same league as us."

—No. Where can I poo?

To my dismay another writer answered.

"The bathroom's over there. In that corner."

My mushroom-addled mind somehow conveyed to me to her core message: she was very pretty, and I was very embarrassed. I began waddling away, hoping it was in the direction she'd pointed.

I must have farted a hundred times in that short stretch. It was impossible not to know it was me. I distinctly remember farting directly in the face of the head publisher, who was unfortunately sitting down in my path. I didn't feel that bad. He had shite taste in poetry anyway. This moment exhibits some of the less cool aspects of mental health. Although, I guess you don't have to be bipolar to eat mushrooms and fart gratuitously.

It wasn't just independent publishing events that I stank up, either. The first time I met Velociraptor, or Raptor for short, was at the International Festival of Authors at the Toronto Harbourfront. Raptor — without giving away too much information, reminded me of a bird of prey. Keen-eyed, sharp-clawed ... a hunter: an apex predator. They were from a different age, a classic age, and they were one of the most celebrated dinosaurs on the scene. I knew of them not because I'd read their work in school (though, I should have), and not because I'd gone to publishing school — I knew who they were because I am a Canadian, for better or worse.

* * *

As an attendant, I get a free notebook in a gift bag. On the way from one event to the next, I notice Raptor sitting next to a stack of books. What luck! Keeper is a huge fan of this writer and would die for an autograph. I approach at speed, directly, and don't pay much attention to the details. I am intoxicated.

—Hey! Wow, [Velociraptor], it's so cool to meet you. Could I get your autograph for my girlfriend?"

"Don't you want my autograph for yourself?"

—Ha, that would be very generous of you, but to be honest, I haven't really read much of your material. My girlfriend is a huge fan, though.

A dull glare meets me, like the stare of a surprised, derisive, Cretaceous carnivore.

"You haven't read my work? How have you gotten through school without reading my work?"

I now realize this author may be slightly full of themself, and I should probably tickle their ego to dig myself out of this hole. My only in, though, is my girlfriend's admiration ... I genuinely know jackshit about Raptor. For fuck's sake, I was the only kid in my school who failed the grade ten literacy exam.

—Umm. I grew up overseas. So, would it be OK to get your autograph? It would make my girlfriend's day.

I proffer the fresh notebook and a pen and curl as convincing of a smile as possible.

"Are you going to buy my book to get it signed?"

Again too late, I realize that this isn't me asking an author next to a stack of books for an autograph, this is me butting in line at a book signing to ask an author to sign an empty notebook. I'm not precisely "in business" at the moment. I buy drugs for myself and a few friends. But my wallet isn't exactly afloat. Think fast.

—I want her to be able to read your autograph and be inspired to fill this notebook with her own writing.

Grudgingly, it seems, Raptor can't compete with this logic and signs the notebook.

—Thanks!

"You still won't buy a book? I'll sign that, too."

—Oh, no. I'm a writer. I can't afford it.

"It's only twenty-five dollars."

Fuck your "only." Whatever, I try another route out of this.

—Look. Truth be told, I have some issues with reading. As I'm getting sicker and sicker, I find I just can't get through a long piece of fiction or creative non-fiction anymore. I can read the news and essays, but whenever I try to read something I want to, I can't help but try to edit it. It's maddening. I could be reading Shakespeare and can't stop trying to make it "better."

Raptor looks strained and bored and, understandably, irritated.

"You yearn to make my writing 'better'? What's wrong with reading for pleasure?"

—No, that's not what I meant. It's just, I'm bipolar, and I'm not entirely certain what that means. But it's getting progressively worse, and I'm losing my ability to read. Which is devastating.

Raptor's eyebrow twitches when I say I'm bipolar.

"Wasn't this meant to be for your girlfriend?"

Shit. I ... umm ... I think Raptor just made their move. And I think they used my own point against me. I name-dropped my mental illness not to explain my failings and foibles, but to get something I don't deserve. And I think that may have pissed them off as much as it would piss me off.

I cut my losses and walk away.

NINETEEN

2017

My mental health journey isn't being made any easier by the absolute and fundamental destruction of modern, conscious social order I'm seeing on the news every night. It feels like I'm reaching a calm point in the stormy seas and can finally send up a flare, only to notice an atomic weapon being tested on not-too-distant shores that moments before had seemed like salvation.

I'm close to being ready to find a job, support myself, contribute to my relationship, even get a fucking dog: I can feel it in the clean, well-oxygenated, well-medicated blood I'm feeding my mind with these days, in place of some pharmaceutical scientists' side projects and secret profit-incentivization motives. I lift weights, do sit-ups, push-ups, and cardio every day. I'm eating as close to healthy as my North American male diet will let me. I'm almost at socially acceptable — and now socially acceptable is slipping into something unprecedentedly palaeolithic for the modern era.

I feel like Marcus Aurelius reincarnated into Caligula's reign. My Wise Mind knows of little wisdom beyond my own mind these days. "Fake news," "alternative facts," "post-truth": How am I supposed to orient myself now? How do "sane" people do it? Is anyone sane anymore? Were they ever?

I need that dog. Keeper and I have a pair of twin male bunnies, and they're adorable, and I love them and their cute little diamond noses and fluff-butts, but they're definitely more her pets; I'm a wolf man, which means I'm a dog boy, for society's sake.

I've had two dogs in my life; only a few months of my life so far has been spent without a dog by my side, and every one of those months has been horrible. I like the feeling that something innocent and pure depends on me and that, as long as I am good to it, it will love me unconditionally. I like knowing I'm giving a creature a good life instead of an uncertain one. I also happen to pathologically require unconditional love from something, largely since I have so many conditions that need to be addressed and dealt with: using love, ideally.

My last dog, Java, who passed in April of 2016, was my girl. When I got her in grade six, my parents phrased it like she was my kid. We made a contract for my responsibilities. I've always wanted children. A legacy, of sorts. I ended up coming to see Java as my kid — more, I think, because of who I am than how my parents approached the situation.

Keeper jokes that she's my woman, but Java will always be my girl. That's true: in a partner I need (for me) inconceivable amounts of inner strength and determination — all the men in my family depend on strong women; but for my furry-friends, I need to see myself as their protector and prime patron. I feel an impossible-to-resist urge to be a parent someday (whether this is a good idea or not, all things considered, might be dealt with in a later chapter), and dogs are like lifelong children. Not to mention, they keep you active and stuck to a schedule, which some people may abhor, but the mentally ill often require in order to give their lives a semblance of regularity. Java was a mutt — a complete smorgasbord of beautiful dog. Whatever mix she was, she was glorious and one of a kind.

She was a street dog until I adopted her the day after she arrived at Scarborough Humane Society. She was about one year old. I saw her online, rushed in, took her out in the test yard — she did her business then fetched a stick for me to throw, only to have her retrieve it and find my inner harmony in the underbrush, bringing it back with her stick and gingerly dropping it into my hand. She was extremely thin back then. All ribs and hips. Not the grizzly-shaped beast I remember her as most, in her older years.

When we brought her home, she didn't understand stairs. She'd fly up them with her hind legs slung low, haphazardly dashing up and down, searching for a foothold. Meanwhile her front legs madly pulled her body up behind her as if she were being chased by gravity personified as a bear. Then once she'd gathered courage again at the top, she'd try to come down sideways, one front paw and one back in each step, like a jackal channelling a crab soul. When we took her to the summer-dry outdoor hockey rink (so we could close the doors, unsure yet whether she'd bolt on us), we only had to throw the tennis ball two or three times before she was exhausted, panting like a great-grandparent doing pull-ups.

Two weeks later she was a shadow dancer. Mostly black, with strips of white on her nose and chest, she seemed to hover off into the distance when she ran, never leaving any feet on the ground, merely tapping it with each paw in a melody only she could hear or keep up with, until coming back dutifully when called to receive her praise and liver-treat slivers. She was my best friend for so long.

She started falling down in her last few months. We'd be walking, and she was mostly blind by then, and she'd just start listing to the left, then her haunch would collapse. Then she'd have a confused look on her face, maybe rub her nose, before looking up at where she knew I was and smiling, tongue lolling out in joy at sensing her boy on the breeze.

One night she listed to the left again, through a baby gate and down a flight of wooden stairs onto a slate floor. My parents found her in the morning, twisted, but smiling to see them, as always. I got the call as I was headed into work, just before I went out of range under the TTC station. Very few things help me believe the world is a beautiful thing, but getting that call in time is one of them. There was no question: I had to be there for her. Fuck the job, if it came to that. She was my world, and she was ending soon. I called into work, The Mercy, a dispensary, and they were compassionate with me, as usual. Someone agreed to come in and cover for me, and I waited for Dad to pick me up, with Java sprawled on a blanket in the back seat, on the way to the vet clinic. I called Keeper and, God bless her forever, she dropped everything and came to meet me. We waited at Bloor and High Park Avenue under the beautiful, foreign spring sun.

When I saw Java, my fundamental manner of relaying thoughts broke down completely. Monkey wrench in the programming of my emotional computing. I've always felt things like joy and security while around animals to a degree that is almost impossible for me with humans. Even my closest loved ones still have to play my mental games to get to me. For animals, there is no charade. I wear one face for all animals alike, all the time. She was yelping, head sickeningly yanked to one side, tongue lolling out with no charm for me in sight anymore. She was covered in vomit and feces and urine from her hours alone at the bottom of the stairs, three flights away from my parents' room and out of yelping range. She was my adolescence, once so proud and fluid, now twisted in upon itself in a crippled and crippling display of anguish.

We finally got her into the vet clinic private room, and the vet spent ten absurd, pointless, and agonizing minutes discussing options for sustaining her life for long enough to say goodbye properly. I almost lost it on the vet, who I'd once worked with while an assistant for this very clinic (my high-school job) — I interrupted her as she was asking whether we wanted a paw print and a lock of her fur, not kindly:

—Just put her out of her pain. For God's sake, give her a dissociative anaesthetic combined with hydromorphone in one injection, wait a minute, then give her a massive injection of Euthanol.

I later felt like an ass for spelling out the vet's own job to her in such blunt language, but my girl was now screaming, her yelps congealing into one long, drawn-out whine, and twitching, worsening her contortions. The vet complied. Something about the veterinary equivalent to the Hippocratic oath must've compelled her to at least do something other than a shitty sales job.

Five minutes later I was petting Java for the last time. She was still. She looked happy to have had our company for these final moments. Just happy, as usual, when she was with me.

```
It's such a slog to wake up and walk
the dog in the morning;
and, a warning: you'll miss it

before long. The minute you notice
your palm isn't licked by 6AM

and you're still storing a leash
attached to a collar with nothing in it.

You'll miss it.

It's been five years and I still get
   puppy dreams.
I miss my Java Bean, and coffee is no
   substitute.
I miss my Beckie, and she died more than
   half my life ago.

It's such a slog to wake up and walk
the dog in the morning, and enjoy it.
```

Losing Java felt like maybe having a kid isn't enough to leave a legacy. It's a biological legacy, sure, but there are so many ways a person, or dog, can imprint upon the world. I remember Java, but who will remember her when I'm gone? You will, now. Same with a kid. Who will remember me when my kid's gone? You will, now. I need to leave a legacy. If not biological, then intellectual, or charitable, or political, or God willing, economic. I need to find a purpose. I need to be remembered the same way Java is in my mind. I want to be immortal. It's not that I'm afraid of death; I just need to play a larger role in life. It's not that I'm doing nothing with my life, either — it's just part of the sickness: I never believe I'm enough, that it's enough. There's no end to this. I need to do better.

TWENTY
2016

Before I get a new dog, I need a job. Otherwise, my dog will be forced to eat something unintended, starting with my valuables, and possibly ending with my extremities. (Not that my parents would let me starve. But I might let myself rather than ask for more help, depending on my future, potential-{hopefully}-alternate-universe mental state.) It feels extremely dirty to me to ask my folks for money. I wonder if the same would be true were I not batshit. It's not that they wouldn't willingly give it to me; it's that something very deep in my gut tells me it's a bad idea.

"Now I'll owe them."

"They'll expect things from me."

"They'll ask what the money's for."

Even if the money's for groceries, I don't like the idea of setting a precedent that questions about my life are OK.

I left The Mercy in June at the time when all the pop-up pot shops were opening in the larger centres of the country. For almost twenty years, The Mercy had been the only player in the game in this city, but suddenly there was competition from every side, from big BC-backed contenders, from *actual* investors, not just crippled hippies with fantastical pipe dreams. The standards and expectations from our member base soared: Why weren't we delivering or carrying this and that rare, already-monopolized-by-someone-else product? Why didn't we have more staff, or stay open late, or open early, or do whatever else a spoiled customer can demand?

I was in the process of moving from server/general cannabist to head extractor/product artist/baker/alchemist. This was a move I was generally OK with, but I knew I would miss the one-on-one experience of budtending — leading a grandma with glaucoma through what to expect after her first puff or nibble off a cookie; hooking the parent of a child with epilepsy up with syringes of the coveted Charlotte's Web, rich CBD oil. It was, generally, a feel-good job. I even got some informal boxing lessons from a patient who'd gone the distance with Mike Tyson in his prime. It was a cool fuckin' gig.

I didn't like the idea of spending too much time in the kitchens, but that's what the management needed: product — high-quality and fast, to stay ahead of the game while they still had a lead. Another factor for friction was the disconnect between my scientific theory, best practice, and standards, and their desire to recoup potential losses, hedge their product gambles, and basically make money wherever possible, without understanding much of the medically verified knowledge I was laying out for them. There's only so much comprehension of biochemistry that a preparatory career as a heroin addict or former convict or retired housewife can provide ... and I just couldn't get certain concepts through to them.

They'd accumulated, over the years, a massive amount of bad bud — mouldy, egg-infested, bud rot, you name it. There were dozens of pounds' worth of examples all over the place, in storage for a wished-for salvage to the investment. They thought I, with my demonstrated ability to make artisanal extracts out of primo product, must be able to work some weed-wizard magic and produce kilos of top-notch hash, or shatter, or e-cig juice, or tinctures, or ... or anything! Anything as long as it worked and did what it had to. The thing is, it would've worked — people would've gotten high, true, but I don't know what else they would have gotten. Even my education in cannabis is limited to what evidence exists: *garbage in, garbage out.*

"Well, can we make hash out of it?"

Granny ran the clinic. She was peering at me from over her exaggerated lime-weed cat-eye frames as she finished licking the glue on a cone the size of King Kong's cock. She looked like Yubaba and acted like Suge Knight. Nobody fucked with Granny. She had family connections to the actual benefactors and ... well ... we were still in the "grey" market, after all. We weren't totally safe from the cops or insured against ill-wishers. We did need some element of muscle.

—Nah. It's junk. Sorry, we can't recoup on this stuff without exposing people to potential hazards. Like, the mite eggs will make it into hash, and the mould would be even more pronounced. People would even taste it. It would be bad for business, too.

I tried framing it in a way they might get more out of: "You might lose money."

"What if we just make edibles out of it? Maybe the decarb process will filter out the bad stuff?"

OG was one of the OGs of the weed game. Tall and lanky, always wearing jeans and one of various neutral colours of plaid button-up shirts, he'd been a pretty heavy-duty skag and bone man for most of his life until he cleaned up with a fuckload of Suboxone during a stint in the infamous Don facilities. He grew a shit ton of weed, semi-legally, on behalf of legitimate medical patients, most of which he sold through The Mercy. It was great stuff. His Cinderella 99 remains unparalleled by any I've tried since. Fit my needs like a glass slipper. And naturally, he knew about the downsides of growing — when a grow goes bad and you're stuck with a few hundred pounds of illegal grass that smells and sells like used adult diapers. He should've known better.

—Maybe, but I can't say for certain. And I'm not willing to try.

They weren't happy. That made me anxious. Pebble in a still pond; I sensed a change in the air.

I just kept remembering what my dad had said when I told him about my promotion to the kitchen: "Don't kill anyone, please." I couldn't guarantee that I wouldn't if I used that trash to make medicine. I quit while I was emotional — never a good idea — then catastrophized my lack of a job into a lack of a future.

I should have just tried talking to them again, made it simpler, negotiated, but I jumped ship. Then once I had nothing to do, I got into trouble again. Add a few months of sunny, dogless days I didn't spend in the park and a side of drug abuse, and I can see why I was admitted to the hospital in late September — but I wasn't admitted voluntarily. I was kept "on form."

TWENTY-ONE

Retrospective on 2016

The emergency ward of a mental hospital is, by definition, not a happy place. The very act of going to emergency can cause people trauma. Being kept there against your choice as you amp yourself up in a drug-induced frenzy to believe that everyone who loves and cares about you was just pretending all along in order to abandon you and have you locked up, potentially indefinitely, and subjected to all sorts of horrifying shit (like forcibly injected medications and all their side effects, which the doctor has time to consider and respect during her five-minute break in the last five hours; cramped conditions with fellow extremely unstable patients; involuntary and invasive medical procedures — it's ugly on the front lines of any war) is absolutely, reality-bustingly terrifying.

Many of my friends also suffer from mental health issues, and one of their stories stood out in my mind while I was in the triage room of the College Street CAMH facility. The Godfather — ten years my senior and with symptoms disturbingly similar to mine, just aggravated (perhaps simply from an additional ten years of this crazy life and subsequently hectic lifestyle, which takes a toll on yòu) — had spent that ten extra years, between age twenty-five and thirty-five, confined against his will in a similar mental "health" facility. Mesh grates on the windows that aren't already permanently draped dark, and bars on all the doors, of which many lead to nothing but more over-filled, perhaps gender or diagnosis specific, perhaps Heinz 57 of madness rat traps, all under the weak and fluttering fluorescent skylights, held to their daily routine closer than that most rational of minds we should all aspire to emulate: *I. Kant.*

I knew a few things for certain during flashes of lucidity amid the delirium of emotion: I didn't want to take any first-generation antipsychotics, many of which have a well-founded reputation for causing more permanent damage than they prevent; I didn't want ECT, or "electroconvulsive therapy," which, granted, has come a long way since it replaced lobotomies as the go-to "option of last resort," but is still known to occasionally alter your personality and rob you of vast tracts of your retro- and anterograde memory functions (I realize there are lots of memories I'd be better off without, but I can't give up Java, or her predecessor Beckie, or my Nain and Taid, or Grandpa before the Parkinson's set in, or the security I felt only in my very early childhood, the memory of which now serves me as a grounding rock ... one of the few things that remains constant in my mind, no matter what) — the Godfather had ECT and didn't speak fondly of the experience or fallout; and finally, I didn't want to be ignored, or left alone, or forgotten about in a room while bureaucratic necessity ruled the nurses and orderlies. I knew, at least, that I wasn't safe with myself in charge.

I sat in the waiting room with my parents, who had taken me in under the pretense of getting checked out, hopefully to get some meds and head back home. There were a few other people in the sterile white rectangular room with its one long window along the wall, reinforced by steel mesh, showing us the staff hustling through our respective files, shooting us dodgy looks. One girl, about sixteen or seventeen, alone and with a tangled mass of brown matted hair, sat on the ground near the door to the bathroom, petting the wall. The petting became more aggressive, mixed with soothing words. Soon she began clunking her head against the bone-white wall tiles. *Thump. Thump.* The clunking became a thunking — what was she thinking? Was she thinking? An orderly came and gently led her to a chair, where she curled in on herself, like a schizotypal kitten. I tried mimicking her, but the chair's arms impeded my ability to stretch out. It was like trying to catch a nap in an airport, and I had no idea when my flight was taking off. A few other distressed-looking people sat in various random chairs around the room, some with family or friends, some alone, some with an orderly standing nearby — all of us stealing glances at each other, judging and empathizing at once. Can't say anyone looked happy to be there, least of all the staff, which only added to my concern. After about an hour the nurse called me in to the screening room and asked me some questions:

"Do you feel safe?"

Obviously not, I was in a fucking loony bin.

—Not particularly.

"Are you worried that you'll hurt yourself?"

Worried? No.

—I don't think so.

"Are you thinking about hurting yourself?

Thinking? Sure.

—I guess so.

A few questions later, I was allowed back out into the waiting room. I sat there with my parents for about half an hour.
Then the two biggest orderlies I'd seen milling about the place
approached me from different angles. They came to flank a
tiny nurse who squeaked out:

"We've decided to hold you on form. We don't feel that it
would be safe for you to return home."

My parents looked worried, but oddly relieved.

I threw my shit in the fan.

I jumped up and bolted to the bolted-shut door leading
outside. I needed a key card. I didn't have a key card. But I
weighed about two hundred and fifty pounds. I took a run
and did my best rugby tackle at the door. If it were a human,
it'd have a punctured lung. But it was a steel door, so I winded
myself. I kicked it as hard as I could. Nothing. I took one last
shot as the orderlies wrestled me into submission. No luck. The
other patients and families, including mine, were ushered out
of the room and I was strapped into a bed and wheeled through
the inner doors. I felt betrayed by the system. I felt betrayed by
my parents. But I'd betrayed myself. The kitten kid looked at
me with pity. Fuck.

It looked like I was no longer in charge of the situation. In
retrospect, I'm glad. I wasn't even in charge of myself.

TWENTY-TWO

Retrospective on 2007

I'm extremely fascinated by mushrooms and fungi — and not for the reason you're probably thinking; though, to be fair, what you're probably thinking *is* likely responsible for this relationship that sees me strolling through forests every spring and fall, searching the underbrush for toadstools and slime cultures. There's no comparison to fresh, wild shaggy manes, diced with onions and crushed garlic, then fried in butter and a bit of white wine, served on a toasted baguette ... but I probably wouldn't know this greatest of pleasures without the assistance of a few small, bluish-bruised, grey-and-brown dried mushrooms that smelled absolutely revolting.

My dad always tried to expand my diet when I was a kid by equating some healthy food with something I was more familiar with. He said mushrooms are just like marshmallows. That they are not, though. This tactic didn't work as well as he'd likely intended. I lean naturally toward a terrible diet. He was right, though — in a sense. I eat more mushrooms than marshmallows now. Maybe he was right about other things, too.

I told him one night while we were driving to get takeout, when I was about sixteen, that I was interested in trying psychedelic mushrooms — purely for therapeutic and experimental purposes. I'd made sure not to have my mom around when I brought it up. To my surprise, he didn't tell me not to do it. He just said something along the lines of, "I don't know much about it. But whatever you do, find out as much about it as you can beforehand, and be careful." I think by then he knew he couldn't stop me from doing certain things; he was just trying to protect me any way possible. I don't know if he even believed I could stray as far as I eventually did.

I didn't take his advice. I'd blindly done acid and mescaline, and a few other psychedelics in high school, but for some reason I'd never tried psilocybe mushrooms until grade twelve. Maybe it's because I'm a squeamish eater, and magic mushrooms are truly nauseating. I know some people can eat them like potato chips, but I gag every time. Throughout grade twelve I tried, unsuccessfully, to trip on mushrooms two or three times before I got it right. Either I didn't eat enough, or they were shitty mushrooms — I don't know. I do remember eating a bowl of macaroni and cheese topped with mushrooms, then passing out immediately after and probably sleeping through my first real mushroom experience. I recall stranger-than-usual dreams, but nothing untoward. So on April 20, international weed day,

I didn't think too much when my friends brought a fat sack of zooms.

I didn't pay too much attention to the dose. After my previous experiments, I had the mistaken impression that mushrooms couldn't be *that* potent, right? And I didn't give smoking huge amounts of cannabis too much thought, being seventeen and it being four-twenty and all. I looked at the proffered handful of alien-looking entities and accepted them like a well-intentioned handshake. This would be a fun night. I put the mushrooms in a cup, pulverized them with a pen, poured in some orange juice, then took the shot. I washed the cup out with OJ and got the last traces into my system. Our base of operations was my friend Tryp's dad's house, but we would be going out on little forays throughout the neighbourhood. That was the expectation. We anticipated lucidity. About thirty minutes after I'd choked down the potion, we set out to a sandwich shop.

* * *

Tryp was the first kid who reached out to me when I went to my second high school in grade ten — that is, the second time I did grade ten. I was sitting alone at lunch, and he invited me to eat with him. It turned out he was just as lost and alone as I was, just more willing to reach out. He was little. He looked like a pale tadpole, and all his clothes hung off him as if he'd lost a shitload of weight; except, he hadn't. His eyes were blank. They didn't give anything away. But he seemed like a nice guy. That first lunch we spent together he got right to the point:

"You smoke weed, bud?"

Was he offering me some?

—Yeah, man. I love weed.

"Me too! Got any?"

Shit. No luck there. Oh well, maybe I'd make a friend.

—Nah. This school is really strict about it, eh?

He didn't seem too concerned about the repercussions of being caught ...

"Yeah. You do anything else?"

—I have.

"Cool, bud. So, wanna chill sometime?"

We became buddies. Friends. I was wary of him, not being able to read him or those cryptic eyes, but I was wary with almost everyone ... so nothing untoward about the friendship stood out. He would, though, become a great trip-fellow. He was into psychedelic literature, music, and culture as much as I was, but he could usually keep his shit together a bit better than me. He was the dependable "sober" one.

* * *

It was a short stroll from Tryp's house in Toronto's Harbourfront to the Quiznos, but it was an increasingly confusing walk. I figured I must've smoked a bit too much or had a strain that was playing tricks on me, as I was stumped by simple things: gates, concrete barriers, signs, etc. It wasn't that I felt entirely fucked; I was just a little lost. A little slow. A little dissociated from my mental faculties. Still entirely present, just, well, entirely present. Stuck in the moment. No focus. Thoughts floated in and out, and while I could sense them, I couldn't make sense of them.

It really hit me in the parking lot. "Hit" doesn't do it justice. It washed and rinsed me in the parking lot. My visual sensibilities became virtual by default. It fucking tie-dyed my eyes. Whoa, this was … umm … googly. My sight was the first thing I noticed, followed shortly by an irrepressible urge to giggle. Everything looked like a Pixar film. Neon reigned supreme. Synesthetic elements crept into my interpretation. I could feel the colours popping out of my palms. I could hear them. I loved it. It was all so strange and sudden, and it took me by storm. I was blitzkrieged by psychedelia, and I surrendered willingly. Reality had been transferred to a digital, downloadable medium, and I was all about it.

—I have Shrek-vision. Everything looks like it's from *Shrek*. Are you guys seeing what I'm, haha, what I'm, hahahaha. Hahahaha. Hahahahahaha.

Tryp countered with irrefutable logic. He was always so on top of any psychoactive situation, but just as reckless as I was, if not more so.

"No way, bud, dude. This is, this is, this is … shit. Fuck me. This is *Toy Story* man. Hehehehehehe. Because I'm *Buzzed*."

I was having none of it. Whatever it was.

—It's all the same company, man. It's … hahaha … it's always the same company. Do you … do you know … what I … mean?

"Don't be a dick, dude. Be nice to people on mushrooms."

Holy shit. I was on mushrooms, and these things were *strong*. I'd always assumed that acid was inherently more intense than shrooms … but that was wrong. Woefully wrong. We walked into the sandwich shop, and I steeled myself for conversation with what were likely sober employees. Talking to straight people when you're twisted is intractably uncomfortable. My turn to order.

—Give me beef. Sandwich. Footlong. Gravy. Chips.

"Would you like some fried mushrooms on that?"

HOLY SHIT! Something here was MEANT to happen. It must've, right? What are the friggin' chances? I could feel neural connections popping off all over my mind like a — like a mycelial network! The mushrooms were speaking to me. All the mushrooms were speaking to me. I was an integral part of every forest, transmitting information and nutrients wherever needed. All of my reality was infused with mushroom essence, like earth had been colonized by an alien life-web alongside a native home-grown life-web, and the two were symbiotic and evolved in tandem but were still somehow separate, and I was closer related to the mushrooms than I was to everything else. The mushrooms made a compelling argument: eat more mushrooms.

—FUCK YEAH I WANT FRIED MUSHROOMS!

Fairly sure the sandwich shop workers were happy to see the backs of us. We went out and popped a squat on a parking barrier to gorge. Those mushrooms burst like juicy fey-land forest-flavoured kernels of delight. How had I never eaten mushrooms before? Mushrooms be dope-swizzy, yo!

We decided fairly quickly, less than an hour after downing the brew — so before they were even peaking — that we were in no condition to be outside, among normals. We decided in hushed whispers in the empty parking lot to head back to Tryp's house and take it a bit easier. We lit a joint (not really fully understanding yet how much stronger psychedelics become when cannabis is introduced) and started the walk back to safety. Out of the corner of my eye I saw — or thought I saw, to the extent that it was just as disturbing as if I'd actually seen it — my family driving by. Oh fuck. My parents couldn't see me like this. I pulled up my coat hood and picked up the pace.

That was too close a call. Close calls are not ideal when dealing with new psychological phenomena.

Back at Tryp's house I went to his fridge, pulled out the milk, and drained the bag. Then I pulled out another milk bag, and drank the whole litre, then went to hunker down on the couch with a blanket and a pillow for what I could tell would be a fairly new, unpredictable, and strange experience. The real visuals were coming in now.

Oozing is a good word for what the 'verse was doing all around me. I contrasted the strange geometric shapes and mosaics, like melting blocks full of squiggles, with the sharp, crisp lines and more grid-like geometry of mescaline and the spirals of LSD, and hypothesized about how the history of regional psychedelics influenced the distinct artistic conventions of certain regions.

Then I remembered Stoned Ape Theory and decided to stop thinking about that until I was sober, since I didn't want to get too deeply ensconced in a pseudo-intellectual, unproven thought experiment, being acutely aware of my momentarily psychedelically susceptible mental processes.

There was no question: I was in a time loop. My first real time loop. And it was horrendous. We'd turned on the TV, back in the days when you'd just watch what was on TV, infomercials included, more than choosing something you actually wanted to watch. But I'd been happy about the *Seinfeld* we were watching until I noticed something funny: I kept seeing the same scene over and over. I looked at my friends to see their reactions, but they didn't seem to notice. Maybe they were dead with their eyes open. How would I explain to Tryp's dad, upstairs right now that, to my horror, I was the only survivor of a batch of poisonous mushrooms. Because that's what these were. Poison. I could feel things inside me. Foreign things. Everywhere. Aliens, instruments, ants. Entities. I was dying. I was losing it. Had I lost it already? Had I ever had it? I wasn't going to come down. I'd challenged myself to see how high I could get, and it was going just like the Challenger shuttle mission. My existence was being spread into the entropic expanse of everything. I was going insane and dying. I looked back to the TV and internalized the *Seinfeld* scene:

"Nothing happens on the show. It's just like life, you know? You eat, you go shopping, you read, you eat, you read, you go shopping ... No stories."

I looked at the clock on top of the TV. It was 8:17 p.m. That couldn't be right. It was 8:17 p.m., like, an hour before. I understood, intellectually, that time could dilate on psychedelics — it had to some degree in previous trips, but never like this. Maybe mushrooms just had a more pronounced effect in this respect? I decided to stare at the clock until it turned over. The clock read 8:16 p.m. *What in the fuck?* I looked back to the TV:

"Nothing happens on the show. It's just like life, you know? You eat, you go shopping, you read, you eat, you read, you go shopping ... No stories."

Ohhh shit. I turned into the couch. This had to be a dream. This couldn't be tripping. This wasn't what happened in waking life. No other psychedelic experience I'd had up to that point could contend. A long ego-ripping dream. As my eyes shut, down came the maroon curtain, and the orchestra tuned their instruments.

The curtain rose to a pitch backdrop. The cast of skulls wearing neon-orange cat glasses and top hats and red capes came down into the aisles to dance for the audience of one.

They spun around me at nauseating speeds, spewing bilious green vapours and mumbling in subaquatic gurgles. Not cool. Not cool. This was a morbid cabaret. I was better off with *Seinfeld*.

I flipped over on the couch, tangled in the blanket and sweating like I was in detox instead of, well, tox. Something's different. The clock broke free. And *Seinfeld* was over. We've cracked past 8:30 p.m.! Now we're watching *Friends*!

Why are we watching *Friends*?

—Can someone change the channel? I fucking hate *Friends*.

"Well, I fucking love *Friends*. Hehe."

I'm pretty sure Tryp is joking and just as reticent about moving as I am, but it begs the question. Who are my friends? Do I like friends? The cast of *Friends* don't seem like very good friends to each other. They lie and cheat and treat each other like shit. Do my friends do that? Do I do that to my friends? Do I just use people?

The mushrooms are my friends.

Tryp's dad comes downstairs as the trip is winding down.

"What happened to you guys? You look like shit."

—Sorry, [Mr. Tryp], I drank all your milk. Thanks for all the milk.

I can't remember the rest of the night ... whether I went home to sleep or crashed on Tryp's couch is lost. What wasn't lost, on any of us, was the significance of the experience. True, there had been terrifying moments. But there was also magic. And it was all natural. Like weed. With thousands of years of human precedent in using psilocybe mushrooms. Maybe these things could help the way I thought. They sure changed the way I thought. I pondered whether mushrooms (with those giggles and childlike wonder) could help me when I was sad.

Or help me discover why I was sad. I mean, I'd taken a load of them and got my head knocked around, but maybe a small dose was the ticket? They would become a staple of my diet. Ideally one I could lean on forever.

TWENTY-THREE

Retrospective on 2017

Part of a new CAMH program I was in (the Transitional Care Program) was nailing a diagnosis. Over the course of four gruelling, multiple-hour interviews, I met with a PhD candidate whose sole function was to get to know me as well as possible, the glory and gruesomeness melding together to form those magical words, my *true name*.

I can't say I wasn't nervous during the final interview. I'd tried to leave no details out — I truly wanted to know who, or what, I am. We explored my criminal past, my family tree, my education and skill set, my dreams and ambitions, my psycho-chemical makeup, and my childhood. She pulled from me as many tears as truths. For someone who tries to forget as much as possible, remembering can be as traumatic as the traumas best left forgotten. But I was steadfast in my dedication. This wasn't for me, as much as it was — this was for my family, my friends, and the woman I love and want to keep loving me.

She began her diagnosis by asking me what I knew about personality disorders. Oh dear. Well, I know that many in the psychiatric community consider them bunk — cop-outs for a more complicated set of symptoms, but I held my tongue. Instead, I said that I knew they were considered more permanent than emotional disorders ... less clear-cut and harder to address.

Everyone more or less qualifies as having some sort of personality disorder, but the severity exists on a spectrum. If it's interfering with your ability to live, it's considered a personality disorder; otherwise, it's a personality type.

Personality disorders usually stem from genetic causes coupled with early childhood experiences, which exacerbate those genes, and as a result, disorders tend to be less responsive to medications and depend more on therapy — retraining the mind how to look at a problem, which takes considerably more time, resources, and effort than a prescription.

She largely agreed with what I said, then continued to tell me that I technically qualify for two personality disorders, based on the severity of my symptoms. The first, and primary diagnosis, was borderline personality disorder, something psychiatrists (at my girlfriend's behest) had already considered for me but had denied pursuing (to my relief), preferring to address the symptoms manifesting themselves as bipolar disorder (type 2) and attention deficit hyperactivity disorder (inattentive type, a.k.a. ADD), both of which were also included in her diagnosis for me.

I was reticent about accepting this name. Everything I'd heard about BPD (mainly through the media and friends) was fairly negative — but what should I really expect for a personality disorder? Good times and groovy feelings all around? I was even less enthused when she pulled up the info sheets to go over with me — approximately 10 percent of BPD patients end up taking their own lives. My tentatively named psychological cohort literally decimates itself. We are also, as a group, so volatile and sensitive that we are largely incompatible with society as it currently exists. Understandably, I was less than enthused with my *true name*.

The second personality disorder I qualify for is antisocial personality disorder. Though, this was less of an exact match according to the information I'd given her. ASPD is the DSM's (that's the *Diagnostic and Statistical Manual of Mental Disorders*) new term for the now defunct diagnoses of "psychopath" or "sociopath." I don't hit all the marks, but enough that it was unnerving to hear from a professional tasked with identifying my underlying persona. I don't feel as empty inside as that diagnosis would entail that I should.

Maybe personality disorders *are* bunk, after all. I hope so, at least. Is denying your *true name* the same as not having one? I don't even believe in magic, except when I'm sick.

Except, I was so very obviously sick. So sick I couldn't see it.

* * *

I graduated from philosophy at university, after spending a few years studying animal and environmental biology, but truth be told, I've never been much of a philosopher. I'm a horrible scholar. I barely read anymore. I used to consume books as voraciously as a flame, but I burned out early, and my memory is ash. I couldn't tell you the difference between Schopenhauer and Heidegger anymore without Google handy. I am, however, a proficient rhetorician. But I couldn't list all the different types of fallacies if you paid me to. They just come naturally.

It was Socrates who said, "He who be a skilled rhetorician has no need for truth."

I can usually dissuade even the staunchest upholder of an idea or ideal. I play the devil's advocate better than the Morningstar could, even without any definite agenda of my own in the act. But I do it to myself more than to anyone else. As a result I have very few core beliefs — more a shifting periphery of values, subject to change as I require them.

The few ideas closest to my foundation, those that shape everything else, I steer my arguments well away from. It's not that I'm absolutely sure of them, more that I'm comfortable with them, and uncomfortable with an alternative, and would rather not undermine the few "facts" I depend on.

I'm a very uncertain person, at heart. When I'm decisive, it's just an act — I don't genuinely know where I'm going or how to get there — I just make it up as I go, the same way I play chess. I still tend to win most of my chess games, but it usually feels hollow. I win because I'm sure of my unsureness, and I inspire unsureness in the surest of my foes.

An old friend I used to play chess with reached out to me today to let me know that another old friend named Lorax died last year. He'd developed an untreatable malignant brain tumour. Two weeks after he found out, he was gone. He never said goodbye. Neither did I. I don't hold either of us to blame for that.

I realized that it isn't only me who can question and annihilate my long-held beliefs. A dead friend can pose the question: "What's the point, if you're just going to die in your midtwenties anyway? What's the point in even searching for a point?"

Is it funny or sad that it takes the presence of death to appreciate life as it is? Is it both? I don't know. I'm not sure: never have been.

TWENTY-FOUR

2009

"What's the point, man? I mean, what's the point of even trying to know what the point is?"

Lorax has this way of questioning even the validity of questioning. His hair, shiny and black, curls into his head so tightly it looks like a toque. He's a bit shorter than me ... maybe 5'10" or so, and "husky," like me. His cheeks are chubby and dimpled, and he looks like a big kid who will never grow up. An American studying philosophy in a Canadian university. Kid's obviously lost. He lives with me now in the house we moved into for our second year at school. He didn't have a place to stay, so we took him in. That makes five of us in the house. He and I play chess all the time. We're about matched, too.

Java takes my distraction at his question as an opportunity to chase a squirrel up an evergreen draped in late winter ice. I let her relish the chase, knowing the liver treats in my pocket will compel her back to my side no matter how swallowed by the darkness she becomes.

We're on a midnight stroll through the park next to our pad and philosophizing as only an undergrad philosophy student and a biology major who aspires to be an undergrad philosophy student can — a few grams of mushroom tea beginning to take hold in each of our already mushy minds.

I've grown tired of studying biology. My early forays into animal biology, with hopes to become a veterinarian, have been trumped by a two-year tenure as a veterinary assistant and the realization that being a vet has very little to do with animal welfare and a lot more to do with swindling customers who believe in keeping their animals around indefinitely to the point that they're willing to part with huge sums of money to keep their already invalid, aged animals alive.

The next step for me was to switch into environmental biology, hoping to save the world from climate change, only to spend two semesters learning from defeated professors about how fundamentally fucked mankind really is.

My early hopes have been rapidly deteriorating into a pessimistic outlook and, dare I say, depression. Despite this tendency toward the negative, the mushrooms are giving me a magical feeling — the sense that we genuinely *can* change the world merely by changing our outlook on it is settling in. I continue with Lorax:

—The point is irrelevant. Well, not irrelevant, just less important. The main issue is the wave that emanates from the point, and how it intersects with the waves it encounters along its way to the shore, the solid.

"How so? Explain yourself, *philosopher.*"

Lorax stretches out the last word to make it clear that I'm at a disadvantage, never actually having taken any philosophy courses, at least not in university.

—Well, think about it, everything has a cause, or source, but how often do we actually nail down that part with any sort of exactitude? Barely ever. We deal with the ramifications of acts and thoughts, the waves. At any given point in time during a rainstorm, you can't tell where the individual drops will fall ahead of time, but by studying the waves in a puddle and how they interact with each other and the edges of the puddle, you *could* track back to the initial points of contact. Or more importantly, you could analyze how the puddle itself *reacts* to those drops, regardless of where they fall, and thereby project forward to future drops, or whole rainstorms, and make contingency plans to deal with the energy distribution, no matter where the energy is *actually* coming from.

"Don't you think that's a bit reactionary?"

—What other choice do you have? Neither of us is psychic, that I know of, at least not yet. You can't tell with certainty where and when that droplet is going to fall, but once it's no longer a droplet, once it's part of the puddle, that's when you can get to work. You can't pre-empt the cause, or droplet, but you can pre-empt the effects of the droplet once you have a general idea of what other similar droplets have done.

"So, even if the cause is random, the effect isn't?"

—It seems random, no doubt, the first time it happens. But it's a big universe. There are no one-offs. Somewhere, at some point in time, it's already happened, or will again, or is happening concurrently to our experience, just a different way.

The snow begins again, covering Java in tiny plates of icing. She's easier to see now, at least, even if it means a more rigorous cleaning once we're home.

"OK, I think I get where you're coming from. But it'd still be nice to know those initial points, and what the point is, don't you think?"

—Sure. Just impossible. And what's the point? We're all part of the same puddle now. We should focus our limited resources on looking at what that means, not why that means what that means.

"I'm not sure whether it's you or the mushrooms, but something is blowing my mind."

For my part, I think that was an exceptionally well-bullshitted dialectic. I don't know whether I made rational sense or not, but I held my ground and defended it, which seems to be what philosophy is all about.

—Java! C'mon, girl. Treat! Let's go home.

TWENTY-FIVE

2006

Tryp's dad is a pharmacist and not entirely opposed to our teenage experimentation. He makes sure we don't do anything stupid. Or *too* stupid. It would be nice to have weed, though, in case I don't feel like using whatever fucked-up stuff Tryp and his dad get for us.

I put thirty bucks in my pocket and take Java for a walk. I call to my parents on the way out the door.

—I might be a while!

"Keep your phone on you."

Yeah. That's the point. Thirty minutes down, and neither of the kids I know who might have pot is returning my calls.

Then … providence! My buddy's little brother, trouble incarnate, and a few of his friends are chilling at the top of the

staircase that leads down to his house. I bet one of these kids
has weed.

Granted, the brother's a few years younger, but he does indeed scare the shit outta me. He's chased my buddy with a meat
cleaver, he collects weapons, and he almost tore off another
kid's nuts with his bare hands.

He looks a bit like a built twelve- or thirteen-year-old Jimi
Hendrix. He's wearing green canvas overalls with one strap
undone and a mock-Rastafarian hat — red, yellow, green, with
fake dreads hanging out the sides. Piece of straw hanging out
the side of his mouth. No shoes. Curious choices. I won't mention any of this to his face.

With some degree of trepidation, I approach.

—Yo, bud. What's good?

He lights up a smoke, then a smile. That could mean
anything.

"Hey, big dude. What's happenin'? How's it been?"

I haven't spoken to his brother since grade eight. Not out
of animosity — we just went in different directions. He likes
sports. I wasn't even sure if this little demon would recognize
me, but he does, and he seems genuinely happy to see me again.
This bodes well.

—I'm good man. Just walkin' my dog and trying to score
some green ... You?

I just kind of leave it there. I'm not asking these tweens for
drugs; I'm just saying I'm looking for some. There's not even an
awkward pause moment — the answer is seamless.

"I got you, bro. How much?"

It's one of the other kids. He's already got his bag open and
his scale sitting on a concrete step. He's wearing all Polo and has
a full left-arm sleeve tattoo. Couldn't be more than thirteen-ish.

—Like, a half-quarter?

"Done."

This was easy. He's fast and they're nice nugs, and he went over by 0.2 grams. Score.

"Forty."

—Oh, I only have thirty.

He looks at my buddy's little brother, who just sort of shrugs. It seems he runs this hoodlum-in-training squad. The kid hands me the bag less enthusiastically than he weighed it out.

"I guess it's already bagged up."

Hahahaha. Keep the change. Mission accomplished, and then some. I ring up Tryp as I walk home.

—I got weed.

"Sweet. I got some cool stuff."

Indeed.

* * *

We're at Tryp's mom's house out in Georgetown. His parents are divorced, and he splits his time between them. Massive house with plenty of spaces to go be alone, and a couple acres of woodland all around it. It's spring and this is the perfect location for what's about to go down.

It turns out Tryp's got a couple bottles of Robitussin, some bottles of Sprite, and a vial of brown stuff labelled as 20X Salvia Divinorum extract. I've never tried any of this shit before, not even Sprite (always been a Coke guy), but he insists they're fun, and I'm down for fun at any cost. This will be a magnificent sleepover.

Two other kids are along for the ride, Buddha and Fuckwad.

Fuckwad's going to abstain from the weirder substances and stick to weed, he tells us. Whatever. He's a mangy mongrel-looking fucker. He refuses to shave his shitty peach fuzz, which only grows on his upper cheeks and lip and is long enough to give him the inkling of a lycanthrope in the making. Regardless, I'll be cordial. I have some sort of inherent respect for fellow psychonauts, even if he isn't doing anything strange tonight. Everybody needs a break now and then.

Buddha is so named for looking like, acting like, and likely being a Bodhisattva. He didn't exactly do well at school … but he had his moments of mental clarity.

We start the night off by smoking a couple of bowls out of Tryp's big glass bong. I don't have much experience with bongs, not allowing myself to have one at home for fear of blowing my cover as a good kid. This is definitely the biggest bong I've hit, and it's got the biggest bowl I've seen yet. Tryp even went so far as to put hot water in it to mix the steam with the smoke, to really get it in there, and added ice cubes to the neck, to cool the smoke for larger hits. I should've one-hit-quit-it, but I seshed hard. I wasn't about to be out blitzed by these guys, Fuckwad especially.

"Maaan, I'm starving. Let's get food."

Fuckwad has a famous appetite. For a skinny kid he sure can pack it in. But I'm hungry, too. The inevitable result of being this high. I can't argue with his logic.

—Seconded. I say pizza.

A cacophony of agreeing:

"Yeah, that sounds good."

"I could pizza."

"Who's calling?"

Ooh. Good question. We are *very* high.

—Let's all call. We'll put it on speakerphone.

This seems like a solid compromise, ignoring that it's a horrible idea. We all head up to Tryp's mom's office, except Fuckwad, who stays behind for a moment to allegedly use the washroom before meeting us upstairs.

"This is Pizza Land, how can we help you?"

Oh shit. We've brought someone else into the circle. Wait, do they record these phone calls for training purposes? What if they can tell we're high and they trace it back to this house? What if the cops come while we're tripping out? How do you deal with cops when you're high? Try being sober now ... NOW. NOW. Nope, not working. What sobers you up? Pain? No, I don't want pain right now. I wonder if the guys are thinking the same thing as me. They must be. We smoked the same weed. Is that how weed works?

"Hello? This is Pizza Land, how can we help you?"

Shit. Shit. Shit. Bite the bullet.

—Hello ... How is your day so far?

Fuck. Mind-fuck me stupid with a shovel, no protection, leaving shards of shovel shrapnel stuck in my skull forever. They know we're fucked. What kind of opener is that? I'm so fucking stupid.

"My day is well. I hope your day is good, too. How may I help you?

—Pizza.

Fuckwad comes upstairs and joins us. Didn't hear a flush ...

"Yes. We serve pizza here at Pizza Land. What sort of pizza would you like?"

Tryp takes a break from chewing his sweater sleeve to pipe up.

"Biggest pizza."

—Yes. Pizza. The biggest.

We're doing OK, I think? Then Fuckwad breaks the scene. "Do you think he can tell we're high?"

We all swivel to Fuckwad and blast him with a flurry of whispers so garbled to our stoned-out ears that probably only the pizza attendant could tell what we were saying, but it amounted to "Shut the fuck up. What the fuck do you think you're doing? Now the cops are gonna come. He's gonna rat us out. You're so fucking stupid."

"And what would you like on your pizza?"

No way. He's in on it. He's pressing the panic button. We should end this call. How do I communicate to the guys not to pursue this ill-advised relationship with Pizza Land without speaking? Buddha speaks, as he does so rarely, with immense gravitas.

"Hawaiian."

I hate pineapple. But I don't want my voice being recorded anymore in case they can extrapolate from the data points composing my voice who I am. I can't give them any more information about myself.

"One party-size Hawaiian. That'll be twenty-eight dollars and twenty-four cents after tax. What's your address?"

No, Tryp, no … don't do it.

Tryp gives him our exact location. Stupid fuck.

"It'll be there in about forty-five minutes. Have a *lovely* day."

The phone line goes silent.

—Buddha, why did you order Hawaiian?

"Yeah, I fucking hate Hawaiian."

"Me too."

He smiles that big vacant Buddha smile.

"I don't like pineapples. I thought being high might make them taste better."

I'm surrounded by idiots. We decide to go get more idiotic off the bong and head downstairs.

—Where's my weed gone?

"I dunno."

"Yeah, bro. No clue."

"Weird, it was right here."

Goddamn it, Fuckwad stole my goddamn weed.

The pizza arrives early. We don't hear the doorbell, being in the basement. Tryp's mom answers the door, pays for the pizza without incident (and, apparently, without Pizza Land ratting on us), then leaves it on the kitchen table. She opens up the door to the basement, and we quickly re-Febreze the room, incense stick sending tendrils from a cherry burning in a bowl of sand. It's OK. It'll take her some time to get down the stairs with her MS.

She just shouts down the stairs:

"Boys, your pizza is here. I'm headed out now. Have fun."

Three of us pick the pineapples off and forcefully eat the remaining ham and cheese glop. Pizza Land sucks. Buddha eats the pineapples and much more than a quarter of the pizza.

—So, you like pineapple after all, eh?

"No, man. That was gross. But nobody else was eating it."

Now it's time to do something new. Let's really get into this shit. Tryp rattles a little glass container:

"You guys ready?"

* * *

Salvia is weird. Straight up.

The classic tryptamines and phenethylamines are hard enough to describe to non-psychonauts, but at least you can compare LSD to 2C-B in a fair few qualitatively accurate ways, and a fellow psychonaut will understand the differences between them through description without actually needing to try both … but salvia is its own beast entirely. There's nothing I can definitively say is like it. And to complicate matters, Tryp has an extract allegedly twenty times as potent as normal salvia leaves, but he bought it from a convenience store, and I don't see any certifications of authenticity on the vial. Just the sun with sunglasses. Why does the sun need sunglasses? Most likely these leaves are just soaked in an unmeasured amount of salvinorin A, the main psychoactive component in the diviner's sage. One way to find out.

We trek to a clearing surrounded by birch trees with polypores sticking off them out back of Tryp's house to get the fully-integrated-in-nature-while-experimenting-with-adulterated-natural-drugs experience. None of us has tried this stuff before. Fuckwad says he has, but he's a compulsive liar, and he says he doesn't have any pointers for us. He's just here to watch. Never fun to have this sort of person around for a sensitive moment. Tryp did some basic internet research; he says he thinks he knows how much to use and insists that the internet deems it "fun." I have misplaced faith in him.

I go first. We brought a little metal pipe and lamented how we'd "lost" the weed to use as a cushion for the salvia. So I just sprinkle a little bit of the twisted brown leaf matter into the pipe and raise it to my lips, with increasing apprehension.

"Dude, you need more."

Goddamit, fuck you, Fuckwad. Calling me out in front of these guys? Like I can't handle it? I double down and basically fill the pipe. With less apprehension, a result of my discontent with and outright anger toward Fuckwad, I level the lighter and spark it up. I'm sitting on a fallen log in pristine nature, and it's beautiful. This might actually be nice. It stings going down, it stings in my lungs, and it stings coming out. Oh, and it tastes like chemicals. I spit between my legs and am surprised by the volume of gloop I hawk up. I wonder if this stimulates your saliva glands.

Ten seconds later I have no space in my head for spit takes. Something seismic is happening. A point of immense gravity has emerged, seemingly from my ass. Oh wait, now it feels like my whole tushie just dropped off into a void. I can feel it, but it's gone. My bum is part of a new black hole singularity centred in my anus. The universe stretches out from my butt and all the light — all of existence, really — is illuminating the objects in the clearing around me, being bent back from its point of origin, my sphincter, to be recycled through my eyes and other sensory organs, then blasted back out my behind to repeat the cycle. Reality and unreality are unzipping from themselves and rezipping into each other. Sheer chaos in colour. Tears open up all around me in the fabric of *is-ness*, and I sense presences emerging from behind them. Ghostly, alien figures. They seem ambivalent to my ingress on their plane of existence.

So here I am. Ass blasting the universe back through my eyeballs, and fucking with zippers that fuck with me right back. This is … umm … something.

Aaand I'm back. It's been about four or five minutes, but it felt like not just eternity, but infinity. I feel rocked even by the abrupt ending, like being jolted by a roller coaster car coming to rest at the end of a wild ride.

"Whoa, bud. Are you back yet? How was it?"

Tryp is eager. I'm too young and naive to tell whether that was worth doing.

—Dude. Awesome. You next.

After a few more minutes, Tryp, Buddha, and I have all had varying amounts of the brown herbs. Buddha sort of lowballed it and said it was weak sauce. Whatever. I know. And Tryp sure as fuck knows. He used even more than me. Fuckwad's disinterestedly kicking rocks, anxious to get back inside for whatever nefarious reason. I guess we're done here. At least we have something else to do now. We'll be Robotripping.

Back at Tryp's house, we pour out the DXM-containing Robitussin cough syrup into glasses, which we then mix with Sprite and proceed to chug as fast as possible, pinching our noses to avoid nausea as much as possible. Tryp had warned that some people throw up on this stuff, but I hadn't expected to feel like throwing up from the smell and taste. We drink a lot. A whole bottle each, minus Fuckwad. Well, aside from the salvia I just smoked, this has to be one of the dirtiest ways I've gotten high so far.

DXM is a dissociative hallucinogen, and it stays true to that description. Robotripping is appropriately named because, if you dare to walk while on the stuff, you feel mechanized, like the Tin Man. You can have synesthesia, amnesia, and full-blown hallucinations, seeing or hearing concrete things that just don't exist. Most classic psychedelics lack this property, and it's something I'm wholly unprepared for. Nausea and an intense feeling of bodily pressure is par for the course with dextromethorphan, but so are other, more disturbing effects ... like time distortions and out-of-body sensations, or physical autonomy, where your body goes about its business without your brain having any input.

I'm noticing a lot of purples on objects with golden halo effects through a very hazy mindset. It's hard to make heads or tails of this experience. Really, I'm just a coconut adrift in the sea right now. Somehow, I'm able to connect with reality for a moment only to hear Fuckwad whispering into my ear about demons and torture and the heat of Hell … stupid motherfucker's trying to ruin my ill-fated trip.

I swing around wildly to smack him but miss and fall down. Time must be playing tricks on me because Fuckwad's not even in the room anymore, but I *can* tell I'm coming down. I decide to go find Fuckwad and give him shit.

Can't find him in the house, but as I pass the garage door I hear the flick of a lighter. Then I smell pot. THAT STUPID MOTHERFUCKER! He snuck out to the garage to smoke MY FUCKING WEED while we were tripping on bottom-of-the-bag, end-of-the-line, desperation drugs. Drug people are supposed to respect other drug people's shit: their trips, their stash, their bodies. Fuckwad isn't a drug person. He's a fuckin' poseur. He just crossed a line, and I no longer have to respect him. I open the door, ready to clock the skinny prick right in the sweet spot of the jaw to KO him.

Fuckwad is prone on the floor in the garage twitching, his eyes darting around, and sort of babbling to himself. The fuck? The air is saturated with smoke, but why's he near catatonic on the concrete? I look a bit closer and see he's dropped something shiny. I try to rub the DXM double vision from my eyes to no avail. I lean closer.

Heh heh heh. Dumbass used the salvia pipe without cleaning it first. I kick him in the gut while he's down and take my weed back, along with forty bucks from his wallet. This was a letdown of a night, but I made a profit, at least.

There are no more rules when it comes to "drug people."

TWENTY-SIX

Retrospective on 2016

The memories from the hospital are hot. They hurt and burn, but also cauterize themselves. They scab over, and the places where those thoughts once dwelled become senseless: not to say they don't still ache, but more as I imagine the ache of losing recollections of a loved one's face. The memories melt themselves.

While I was in the hospital I kept a record of what was happening. When I got out, as I worked on myself, I worked on the record:

```
College St. ACU

    i

"Welcome to the cuckoo's nest,"
```

Maria says, its best-dressed guest
in a sort of meta-trope, the day before
she keeps me awake with her shower song
composed of Russian minor notes

"This place is for broken people," says
    Dillon —
though all I hear is a mumble evoking
    that interpretation

We're all on form; and this was
written with contraband paper and crayon

Today, Tania woke me gently with her
left hand on my leg, until she was wrestled
back to solitary, where you get your own
    TV, toilet, and bed straps

No remote; I can't blame her

She sang me Beauty & the Beast
whatever her intention
        I need to leave

        ii

We have no windows or music or exercise
    or escape

        I stick to myself
I'm not in league with the touchers —
    the feelers
I shower under supervision once a day —
in the same manner I brush my teeth, but
    twice
        I return everything

My girlfriend and family bring extra
    meals in shifts;
they balance three squares, it's hos-
    pital food but I need it,

an involuntary doubling down
on olanzapine and abstaining from
    Concerta, Trintellix, and Abilify —
and the other stuff

I'm not sure whether I'm still technic-
    ally in withdrawal,
or just experiencing the initial symptoms
that provoked my being medicated: I
    exhale
with nothing to inhale; we truly are the
    cuckoos,
I think, watching myself
with only a clock

        iii

Each morning my shoulders are peeled
free, rotated, and reapplied with nico-
    tine patches;
the mentholated cartridges
they give us do nothing
but freshen your breath

        iv

I'm not getting my meds
I get all sorts of meds, but they're not
    mine

When they do, eventually, start
slowly with some daily prescriptions
they introduce them piecemeal,

they are not the good ones

I fake getting better, and in doing so am
getting better — just worse for the
    experience
More wary: no trust

I was individually monitored until I
  tore a strip
off the thin bedsheets and tried to hang
  myself

earning a CODE WHITE, which stands
for aggression — my second — new
  bedsheets
came with the beginning of a tear already
  there
    I noted

    v

All anyone here asks or cares about is
  when they can leave
and what they can get or expect until
  they do

There are no answers, just unstamped pills
to quell the questions
When your form expires, there's a form
  for that

The phones can't dial 911

Sheng, the manic Micronesian kid, is too
  much
for me right now
They offer an Ativan and a loxapine —
he haggles them down to one or the other,

—The red pill will take you down the
  rabbit hole

He pops the loxapine based on that

I establish dominance in the ward
I ask for blues I know are Ativan
on regular, strategized cues,
and only take loxapine at night,

```
and then rarely — only if
    I really need to sleep

    vi

I have an uneasy truce with Dillon
he's more like me than the others
just bigger and non-verbal

Dillon, when you're done in there,
come stay in my spare nowhere

I hope your tongue has shrunk back to
    speaking size by now
Keep on with your Māori chest-thumping —
    prop to lock —
it's what you need to do ·
even if just to stop Sheng's incessant
    chatter

        I get it

Keep your finger on Clinton and Trump
    and the camera in the corner
across from the TV
Keep your finger on the controller, if
    they let you
        have it again

Click "29" and dance,
Dillon, if you're still inside —
even if you're not watching,
just feel it and dance

    It's the pulse from outside
    keep the ward safe for now
```

* * *

I can't read that poem without another part of me melting.

TWENTY-SEVEN

May 1, 2017

Another happy day outside the hospital, and I feel another set of healthy check marks march on by. I'm eating, sleeping, taking my meds … I've been going outside and looking strangers in the eye, even if unwillingly. Happy Calan Mai, my friends! That's the Welsh form of Beltane, the Celtic fertility festival at the turning of the seasons from frost to flowers. The cherry blossoms are blooming in High Park, but I avoid them on the walks to and from my parents' house, south of the forest, due to the rapacious crowds of selfies-with-flowers seekers that swarm our neighbourhood a few weeks every year. I'm still too fragile to creep through that tangle of humanity, despite it causing me to miss out on the delights of Toronto's closest attempt at nature. And at the nicest time in the tides of temperature, too.

I'm still fresh from my most recent trip to the CAMH wards. General Psychiatry Unit this time, like last time in January. Unlike the first time, in September, way back before I started coming voluntarily. Back when I was still being restrained and forcefully medicated. I feel wiser now since I started facing my fears ahead of their inevitable victories and admitting myself to the hell of a mental hospital visit while retaining agency, if poorer for the wisdom.

Another unprecedented week, this time brought on by apoplectic anxiety so overwhelming I felt physical sensations manifested as nerve endings clawing their way out of my stomach, through my skin, my psyche using my entrails as launch pads intended to be burned during liftoff to somewhere safer (like the perpetual silence of suicide). The source of the anxiety was, the doctors and I agreed, a combination of an increase in a mood stabilizer known to cause anxiety as a side effect and completely surrendering nicotine (which has an inhibitory effect on many psychiatric medications) — so essentially, by giving up nicotine, I poisoned myself on lurasidone, the acute repercussion of which was unbearable anxiety. Sometimes the side effects are indistinguishable, or intertwined, with the symptoms. As Paracelsus said, the dose makes the poison.

The ward itself was almost unchanged since January — same dour nurses focused more on paperwork than social work, same "food," same overtaxed doctors who might be able to spare you a couple minutes to talk, maybe tomorrow, maybe. Even a few of the same patients. I'm not sure whether our discrete visits just so happened to overlap or whether these people just never left. I didn't ask them. I wasn't there to make friends. Not this time, with these symptoms.

The anxiety felt like digesting broken glass and razors, washed down with vinegar and lemon juice. My mind was shanking me. Involuntary psychosomatic seppuku. No capacity to write an accompanying peaceful haiku. I couldn't stop pacing the halls or my bedroom. Keeper brought me a stack of books. I noticed I couldn't get past page one on any of them — I even tried *Harry Potter and the Philosopher's Stone*, which I once could've recited by memory. No dice. I stopped trying. When the attendants weren't looking, I would relieve my perceived stomach pains by smacking my forehead against the wall as a distraction; when they were looking, I'd grab some skin and pinch it. I knew well enough not to be sent back to the ACU for self-harm. I couldn't sleep or eat or stay immobile for more than a millisecond until I was convinced to take some lithium and benzos. I'd been unwilling to try lithium, due to reports I'd heard of it being associated with liver damage, given that I've already done so much damage in that area, but the doctor made a compelling case:

"It might help."

I was terse in my response. I'd barely spoken to anyone during my tenure there, overwhelmed by cognitive distortions: catastrophizing my latent black-and-white thinking and emotional reasoning into mind reading, jumping to conclusions, overgeneralization, and personalization. My mind felt like it was being physically tugged in different directions. My third eye was going through experimental laser surgery, and I felt warped in totality, somewhere between Leonard Nimoy and Pete Doherty, like the entirety of me was in one of those photo filters that enlarges certain parts of your face like a funhouse mirror. The nuthouse is not a fun house, though.

Fuck it, I thought. My guts were already being shredded.

—Fine.

That's one admission for psychosis, one for depression, and one for anxiety in the last six months, each with aspects of the others as well. I seem to be on a roll. Downhill.

I've had a consistent level of ambient depression going on since before my first admission, but I've noticed it becoming more aggressive with each passing day — sort of racing those healthy milestones I'm hitting, in contention for possession of my outlook on life, or something. Sure, I'm taking my meds and exercising a bit, going outside occasionally, but there are a lot of things I can't do.

"Do you think you can make it today?"

My dad doesn't have any trace of accusation in his voice: it's a simple question.

—I don't want to depress anyone. I feel like I'll bring everyone down.

"It's a funeral. He was seven. Everyone will be crying."

A young boy I knew, Innocent, had strayed on his bike from a pedestrian path into oncoming traffic several days before. Another white bicycle on the road.

—I'll be crying for him, too. But I'm still crying for me.

I remember Innocent knocking on our door while passing through the neighbourhood, just to see Java and say hello. He loved her and she loved him. Mutual innocence. He couldn't compute negative thoughts. I don't think he was capable. He was special to so many people. It's going to be a big funeral. I don't have the wherewithal to look his family in the eye and reserve any of my sadness for myself. It feels traitorous to his memory.

—No, Dad. I'll stay here.

"We'll give our love to his family for you."

Yes, please.

Then they leave. I feel very cold. Very, very cold. I start shivering and coughing and crying and hitting myself and drooling and screaming and rolling on the floor. I am not a professional mourner; this doesn't look practised.

I need to get better. I want to get better. I deserve to get better (maybe not, in all fairness, depending on your cosmic sense of justice, but I have to say it to believe it, and I have to believe it to understand it, and I have to understand it to get it). My sister's home. My nephew's home. My family is back together. It's been so long. Almost ten years since she moved to the UK. I thought our little team had been split up for good, but now she's back, and she brought more family!

* * *

One Saturday we all go to the St. Lawrence Market in downtown Toronto. Free-sample day. Me, my parents, my sister, her partner, and my nephew. I carry the little guy in a BabyBjörn while he occasionally sneezes in my face between hugs and squeaking out:

"You my best big buddy."

I love every moment of it. After the market we go for dim sum on Spadina. The waiters come by with carts covered in bamboo steamer baskets, and my nephew eats almost as much as I do. Three generations of us at a round table, just digging in — barely talking until we all sort of lean back with the dim sum–itis. My dad drops his standard line at this point:

"It's all the water you drink. It just blows up the rice in your stomach until you feel like bursting."

No shit, Dad. We all know. But we also all love how he always repeats himself, telling the same story over and over, even after you interrupt him to tell him that you've heard the story a million times. His dad did it, he does it, and I do it.

We're a family again. But there are still strains. I spend a lot of time on the couch, crying. My nephew is three:

"You sad, Uncle?"

—Yes. But it's OK. It's just a passing part of life. I'll be better soon.

I have to prove it. I can't let him watch me fall apart on a couch. I can't expose him to the viral load of my mental illness. I can't lose myself again, or I lose them with everything else that I am. I have to be a good uncle. I have to be a good brother. I have to be a good son. I have to be good.

To that end, I'm on some new medications and have reintroduced an old one that seemed to work well before. And I'm trying to eat healthier than ever before. The psychiatrist recommended the potential of ECT (my big no-go area) after I got out of the hospital, to deal with persisting anxiety and suicidal thoughts (if not plans), but I declined his offer — I need to know myself, which is hard enough through the drugs, and I'd have to imagine harder after having electric shockwaves pulsed through your brain.

I have Valium to help with the anxiety, and lithium to even out my moods, and escitalopram to elevate those moods, though the latter two will take a few weeks to kick in fully. Until then, it's still a struggle to wake up every day. My eyes open to incipient anxiety, my mind begins repeating nonsensical sentences and half-remembered pop songs, and I start rolling over and over to ease the discomfort in my stomach that is concocted by thinking about the tasks of the day ahead. But over the course of the day, and more and more as each day rolls by and the medications pick up their slack, I begin to feel better. I'm finally starting to feel human again. I hope, desperately, that this lasts. I even smiled today. I made a joke. I laughed with someone else. I'm still depressed as fuck, in general, but that was one of the happiest moments of my life so far: remembering hope.

TWENTY-EIGHT
August 7, 2017

The pace of change is a heartbeat. There are only so many steps an individual can take.

I'm living with my family again. The Keeper situation hasn't worked out as well as planned/anticipated/hoped. To be honest, I don't know why ... well, I know, but only in bits and pieces, not as a whole. The entire reason, in this case, is more than the sum of its parts — and I'm just a small part. I don't feel like dwelling on this point for too long, as the events are fresh in my memory, like a leaking laceration. I'll wait until the scabbing starts to get my hands dirty again with reminiscences; maybe I'll come back to it in a later chapter. Anyway, I'm a single soul again now. I can autonomously revise and reconstruct my persona and hopes and direction again before the next mind-meld.

Other things have changed. I dropped out of my CAMH therapy group. The rules of the group were pretty simple: don't put each other down, don't expose each other to bad influences, get permission before you approach each other in public, and don't talk about self-harm ... it's triggering.

I was doing really well. The group liked me (class clown), and the moderator appreciated my insights — even if my jesting was a bit of a distraction. My mood was up and down. Some days I was hyperactive; others I was depressed. I was never exactly flat. One day I was particularly down. I'd been having suicidal ideation all morning and needed to talk to someone about it. At the beginning of the group, we went around and updated each other on our lives and how we were feeling.

—I don't feel good.

The therapist gave me a sensitive, understanding look.

"Can you tell us more about that?"

I shouldn't.

—I'm having thoughts. Bad thoughts.

That should've given her an inkling to wait till after the session and pull me aside, but:

"What kinds of bad thoughts?"

—Suicide.

Her lips clenched.

"Can you come outside with me?"

We left the group and went into the "quiet room," where I was surrounded by the art of grateful patients, the knitting of anxious patients in search of a mindfulness activity, half-finished sudoku puzzles, Zentangle, mandala colouring books, a keyboard, and an out-of-tune guitar. I'd spent more than a few hours in this room during previous outpatient visits. It had good vibes.

She shut the door.

"You know you're not supposed to talk about self-harm in group."

—You asked me what I was thinking about.

"I have to call you an ambulance if you mean it."

Maybe she wasn't so understanding.

—I can't go back to the hospital.

"You can't hurt yourself. What's more important?"

I weigh my options: hospital, or the devil I don't know yet.

—You don't need to call an ambulance. But I'd like to take the rest of the day off.

She looked at me very closely. I plumbed the depths of emotionlessness and turned off from feeling, if just for a moment. I poker-faced my way out of a tear. I deserved an Oscar.

"All right. I'll see you on Thursday. I hope you feel better by then. Call emergency services if you feel like … like doing something."

When I got home, I dropped out. Probably not a wise move, but one made emotively. And as much as I sometimes hate my emotional vacillations, they do demand a certain amount of respect — they are the antithesis of reason and provide a counterbalance to my constant and occasionally ruthless self-design by means of Occam's razor. I've also decided to revisit the possibility of ECT, and I met with specialists about a month ago. It was decided that, as of now, I'm not a suitable candidate, as I appear to be in remission, but if the situation goes sour, we may need to have a more involved conversation. Better than suicide, I've come to suppose, at least for other people.

On a more positive (or promising) note, I took a much more active interest in my physical health, realizing over the course of the year the full import of its impact on mental health. I tried to get to the gym about five times per week, and noticed significant improvements in mood, energy, motivation, stamina — basically everything that helps a sick person get better. Not to mention the confidence/ego boost of having people tell me I looked sharper, healthier, stronger, and all in all better, which doesn't exactly hurt. I quit cigarettes (and nicotine) completely, only using cannabis about once a week, and barely touching the harder stuff. I'm very, very proud of that.

Living with the family has perks, too. No rent. More space. Company. My nephew is threatening to take my shadow's job, which I fully welcome. I love the wee Fenian monster — everyone says he's exactly like me at that age, and we both get called by each other's names accidentally at least once a day — the cynical side of me, though, can't help but hope that his similarity to me is merely superficial: I wouldn't wish my mind on him.

* * *

I'm writing this at home, sitting across from another competitor/prospect in the small Toronto writing community. I'm reintegrating with society. When I'm sick, I restrict myself to my closest friends (none of whom are writers) and my family: that I'm connecting with other *artistes* and attending public functions again is an excellent sign. I'm even doing a bit of *free*lance editing for a local poetry micro-press — full on immersing myself in the creative game as I can only do when I'm within about 80 percent soundness of mind. You need to be sharp and present with these literary fucks — one misstep and it's like pissing yourself in grade three: immediate pariah status.

The other guy just left, and, as a result, I've given up on writing any more today. I guess, while I might be getting better due to exercise, family, and maybe even my new-found "single status," I'm still not cured. I'm in a sort of psychic limbo.

Cured is the wrong word. I know that won't happen. But I'm still not the "Me" I need to be.

TWENTY-NINE

2013

Something I've noticed about many of the psychonauts who surround me, using the same substances and living in the same world, is their alacrity in subscribing to conspiracy theories. It doesn't take too much prying with many users of psychedelics before you come across something that just sorta doesn't jive with (and they'll hate me for using this word) *reality*. It runs the gamut from fully fledged "some people are aliens and they communicate secret, indescribable messages to me" to "scattering these crystals and their positions, in coordination with the stars and planets, will give you insight to your future." A lot of psychonauts, in essence, are heavily swayed by magical thinking. Whether this is caused by the drugs themselves or is representative of the underlying personality traits present in the sorts of people who seek out further magical realism with the medicines of the gods, I don't know ... but the drugs probably don't help.

* * *

Taking psychedelics, or dissociatives, or stimulants, or opioids, or entactogens, or any other class of drugs is one thing; taking a few together can be something else entirely. Some substances don't seem to interact at all, but some are bad. Some, though, can be a lot of fun. Ever notice how much coke there is on the top lid of every dive bar's toilet? Or speedballing (mixing opiates and cocaine), the chosen mode of exit for John Belushi, Chris Farley, and Mitch Hedberg. I wonder if it's the comedy that got them.

Tonight I'll be mixing a new concoction, a cocktail I haven't tried before. It's well past midnight, and I'm at my parents' house in Toronto. I have to be very secretive. They went to bed hours ago, but I've waited a bit longer than usual because, well, I don't know what's going to happen. Luckily, it's a big house. Secrets can be kept here. I dropped a tab of good, clean acid about forty-five minutes ago, and I'm preparing the next ingredients in this recipe. In front of me are a few pre-rolled doobies and three pencil-thin but long lines of ketamine: the nice stuff, the stuff that looks like shards of glass and stings like peppermint — the pharmaceutical supply. The last ingredient is the sketchiest-looking item on the table, though. A bowl pipe with about thirty to fiftyish milligrams of N,N-DMT — it's hard to measure accurately, so I'm going by look.

I vanish the first line in one go, then hesitate for a second before rashly snorting half the second line, suddenly stopping midway through when reason tells me to quit while I'm ahead. Compulsive redosing is just a feature of ketamine. And as should be abundantly clear by now, I have difficulties reining in my baser instincts. I'm not a big fan of K-holes, but I do enjoy a nice moderate dose. Like all the best parts of being drunk without the hangover. It also has a slightly psychedelic vibe, especially as the LSD begins working its magic on my mind.

I lay back and put on Funkadelic's "Maggot Brain" and cozy into myself for what feels like hours, but I know by now it is only really minutes. I contort under the blankets that have appeared on me from wherever, or whomever. No … wait, I'm alone. I did this. My short-term memory is bunk right now. I look at my watch: I'm an hour and a half into the acid trip. The peak is coming. I spark up a joint, careful to exhale the smoke up my parents' chimney, and let it coax even more psychedelia out of the tryptamine.

It's time for the next step. I raise the bowl pipe to my mouth and begin heating the contents with a lighter, careful not to touch the flame to the glass. Soon the crystals melt and begin bubbling, the vapour begins curling in the confines of the orb, and I place my lips on the mouthpiece and inhale long, and deep, and slow. The powder has turned into a brown resin clinging to the bottom of the bowl. There might be a bit of trip left in there, but I got the majority of it. I exhale in a rhythmic fashion, exhaling a small amount and breathing back clean air, exhaling a little, then inhaling, keeping the vapour inside me as long as possible. After about ten breaths, I exhale long, and deep, and slow. The room fills with grey-white steamy-looking particulate matter clouds, layering like there's a storm in the forecast.

Something like a gong goes off as I rock back on my butt to lie facing up to the ceiling, which begins doing very strange things for a white, stucco ceiling. I hope my parents didn't hear that gong. I'll be out of commission for a while. This will be one for the memory books.

As I mentioned, my short-term memory is a bit finicky already. But several things fundamentally more disconcerting begin happening, all in concert. I am in a dissociative, tempestuous cartoon land, and it may be too much. We shall see. Too late to do anything about it now.

My long-term memory is short-circuiting. Flop. Blop. What's my name again? Where am I? What is *is*? I have no ability to remember anything whatsoever. I am absolutely at this point in the grips of ego death. I don't recognize *I* as a construct. There are inputs being entered into my mind, but there's no witness here. Nothing is happening upstairs. I am at the mercy of nothingness, and nothingness is not reciprocating the arrangement. This feeling lasts for a subjective infinity of what is likely approximately two or three minutes before oblivion releases its hold on me and I'm *me* again. Yay me!

The next stage of the trip, the comedown, if you will, is still as intense as the first part. I wander hallways composed of hallways, chock full of hallways, like a much more convoluted version of M.C. Escher's *Relativity*. These are layered in an interlacing six, or seven, or eight, or eleven, or however many dimensions there are, or seem to be, gigagon-grid layout. One door with a looking glass peers into a study full of books and globes and parchments and Da Vincian inventions, and I open the door into what turns out to be a portal of some sort into strange space. I step into the space oddity and gravity immediately dissipates. First I lose sense of the floor, then my clothes seem to be drifting loosely. Unnervingly, my muscles and skin start falling off the bone like perfectly done ribs. In no time I am losing molecular cohesion. There is no connection between what were the parts of me and anything else. The vast, vast majority of all space is taken up by emptiness. I fall apart at the subatomic level and homogenize with the fabric of gluons and quarks coalescing around pockets of pure, radiant energy. I become nuclear pasta and am squeezed as near as possible by a sudden rush of gravity into a singularity, stopping short as a neutron star. I live out the life of a neutron star until I burst, again spreading my essence into nothingness. Gradually I reconvene myself into, erm, myself. First I gather as chemicals, then those chemicals undergo a set of processes to become molecules, then cells; then born from a dead star, I begin to hurtle like an asteroid recombining into humanoid shape and am rocketed back to the ottoman I'm lying on, still faceup, slack-jawed, and with a brain as emptied out as the result of a well-aimed drive-by shooting. I open my eyes and the white stucco is back to doing the relatively more normal stuff it does when you're just on acid and ketamine. There are tears running down my cheeks. The whole experience probably lasted about five minutes. They call this the businessman's trip, but to me it's five minutes of forever.

* * *

I can certainly see how other psychonauts would take an experience like this to a mystical place. Possibly to a dangerous place; charismatic leaders like Jim Jones have been known to use drugs to make their accomplices more suggestible. But hopefully, there aren't too many of them around. People like

Timothy Leary, though, arguably did more harm to the cause than good. Fuck Joe Rogan. We need fewer psychedelic evangelists in this community and more fact- and research-based science. We need to really get to the bottom of what these chemicals can do for you. Because I feel fucking fantastic.

THIRTY

Late Spring 2012

I've been home about a month or so, back with my folks, and we're driving each other barmy. I'm on probation, so no drugs for me. I'm living off of tobacco smoke and a new barrage of medications. Only natural to chafe with your adult child living back in the nest; all the more so when they should probably rightfully stay in prison. Still, my folks are being as gentle as possible. But I need someone my own age to chill with. Or more to the point, someone like me.

"I ran into [the First Man]'s mother tonight up on Bloor. She said he's back from university and he sounds as pent up as you do."

The First Man, or "the Man," is the first kid I met when I moved to Canada. He was tiny. Just friggin' tiny. We'd gotten

back from Jersey in the spring of 1997, then spent a few months
in a hotel overlooking Queen's Park while our house was reno-
vated — in anticipation of having kids once again running
through the more than a century–old house. I was eight on the
first day of school that September. He was standing there out
front of the portable we'd been assigned to, and I went over and
introduced myself. He seemed friendly, and he was. He lived
nearby. That's enough for eight-year-olds to be friends. His
mom was a hippie psychiatrist, his dad was a hippie scientist,
and my parents were both straightlaced number crunchers. We
were tight for a few years, then gradually drifted apart. Going
to different high schools was the final nail in our adolescent
relationship's coffin. Still, he was the first kid I smoked with,
so he's in my memories for that, at least.

We were nine or ten, and it wasn't weed or tobacco. His
Jamaican nanny had taught him how to roll for her, so set loose
in his mother's backyard, we would roll up mystery plants and
smoke them on our lunch breaks. I highly doubt that he's as
pent up as I am.

"We thought it would be nice if you two went on a bike
ride, like when you were younger. Why don't you call him? I
know he'd probably like to get together, too."

The fuck? Am I going on an organized bicycle date with my
childhood buddy as my first social foray after my brief incarcer-
ation? Umm … I guess I have to. I don't pay rent or anything.
Good behaviour is all I can offer.

—Yo, is this [the Man]? Yeah? It's me, yeah. My mom says
she ran into your mom or something? Yeah? Umm … I guess,
yeah? So … do you wanna ride bicycles with me?

I'm twenty-two and this feels ridiculous.

"Yeah. I guess I could ride my bike today."

—The lake?

"Meet you at the bottom of your folks' street in fifteen."

—K.

This is gonna be weird. I haven't spoken to this guy in about ten years. I bought weed off his brother once or twice in high school, but I have no idea who the Man has become or what he does. I'm not expecting much. I don't remember enough about his personality to even guess at whether he may have developed into an interesting person or not. I remember not being invited to one of his birthdays and just sort of forgetting about him after that. He likes sports. Fuck him anyway.

I get to the bottom of the hill on my parents' street and see him waiting for me. He's gotten bigger. He's a man now. I wonder if he's thinking the same about me. I remember a weenie little dude six months older but reasonably smaller than me back in elementary school, but he's grown. He's about my height, with a mushroom cloud of tight, tiny dreads squished down and poking out from under a Detroit Red Wings cap: sticker still on. It makes him look substantially taller. This is his helmet. He's rocking a Red Wings jersey, too, but his sleeves are rolled up in the warm late spring midday sun to expose a Zentangle sleeve of intertwining black tattoos reaching up both arms and ending ... well, he's wearing shorts and there are tatts down there, too. I guess he likes the Red Wings — then I remember his dad was from Detroit. He'd moved here in the early seventies so as not to be forcibly relocated to Nam. I feel like he had a moral objection to torching innocent villagers. He towered over all of us and looked and acted like Gandalf the White.

The Man's dad died when we were kids. It was shortly after we'd sort of drifted apart. My dad told me about it and said

I should reach out to say I was there for him. I'd thought it would be an awkward conversation, so I didn't. I was just a kid. I didn't know better, yet. His dad was an awesome dude ... I just didn't say so. He's memorialized in more places than just this book. He was an integral part of our community.

Looking closer at the Man's tattoos, which just sort of blend into his background skin tone, I realize they're pictures of a city, of a man, of words: love, dad, Detroit.

—Yo.

"Yo. Nice bike."

It's gonna be one of those conversations: *What have you been up to? Do you have a girlfriend? What'd you study at university? Etc.*

"Do you drink?"

Or not.

—Yeah ...

"Wanna lock our bikes on Bloor and get fucked up?"

—Dude. I thought this was just gonna be a lame-ass bike ride.

"Man, fuck that shit. I haven't had a beer since, like, ten this morning."

Damn, he's The Man. OK. I can roll with this. We sit down on a patio and watch the world go by, gradually getting blurrier and slurrier. We talk about the old days and what's happened since then. It's a nice afternoon, made all the more choice when a group of kids a few years younger than us stop by our table to give the Man props for being a cool big bro. These are the minions of the Man's younger brother. Some of them are familiar from around the neighbourhood. The Man makes introductions all around. They seem somewhat nefarious. One of them leans forward.

"You want anything, I got it."

—What would I want?

Another pipes up.

"Whatever he don't got, I do."

Interesting development.

—Can I have both of your numbers?

I doubt this is what my mom had intended when she organized my bike date with the First Man. My dad uses biking to stay healthy. He'll bike to work at six in the morning, then bike back well after the sun's gone down before making us dinner. All year long. Canadian winter included. It's his antidepressant. On weekends he'll wake up at five so he can bike to another city and back. Basically doing a stage of the Tour de France as a morning constitutional. He'd gotten my bike tires filled with air and my chains oiled in preparation to come out today. He's so happy to have me getting some much-needed fresh air and seeing an old friend. A ride is exactly what he would need. But meeting these sketchbags is exactly what I want.

THIRTY-ONE
November 2011

"[Juice] has a proposition for us. It's pretty out there, man. I think you'll go for it."

Chud has this way of always taking on the zaniest projects and assuming I'll be game. It gets us into trouble, but it also makes for a more lucrative return on investments than the safe bets I tend to stick to.

Chud had been one of my lieutenants, grabbing about a quarter of a pound of weed at a time, but within months he was buying in amounts that I couldn't put up the capital to grab on his behalf. I promoted him to full partner of our little firm. He's ten years my senior, but we click like brothers. He likes to say that he's the general and I'm the president, and that's how we'd structured our organization early on. Chud finds people of interest: he makes connections with cops, bikers, townies, professors, and other drug dealers, on and off campus; he networks. Chud brings the proposals. I make the projections. I weigh the pros and cons. I pull the trigger on big decisions. The roles fit our respective personalities, and our personalities complement each other: hell-bent on living for the moment.

—A crazy idea from [Juice]? Shit, I know you're about to say something fucked up.

A bit of context here. Juice is a normal frat dude through and through. We buy high-grade weed off him when the supply from Toronto gets low. His prices are high, but his product is primo, and it all comes from a tight-knit community of hockey-playing, backwards trucker hat–wearing dingleberries. He isn't prone to having unusual contacts or materials, or plans.

We're roving around the city making deliveries, simultaneously a great and terrible part of the job. A) You get out and about and meet old friends and new, interesting people, and B) you're sitting on a large amount of a pretty high minimum-sentencing set of substances. Each of us has a smoke going. He's rockin' Belmonts, like a smooth criminal should, but I'm hackin' Camels, 'cause marketing gets me.

"So, get this man, you're gonna love this. Supposedly, a sub went down in the St. Lawrence River and it was full of Afghani gold-seal hash. Mazar-i-Sharif. Has a fuckin' AK-47 stamped on each brick. Word leaked and [Juice]'s friends' friend's friend had some scuba gear and went down and took some. He took way too much, though, and he's looking to unload some, and [Juice] says he doesn't need that much."

Juice doesn't need that much? How much fuckin' hash are we talking here? I saw a campus security car drive by; we were in Chud's Mercedes, down by the river, a few kilometres from the school. What were they doing over here? Was I too suspicious? Not suspicious enough? I dunno. I've never really done this before. Not at this scale. Every day's a new adventure. Every lesson is a pass or fail with grave consequences.

—What does it cost?

"That's the thing. Buddy only wants to do one deal with one person, or in our case just the two of us. Get it all done at once, y'know?"

Red light. Pedestrians start crossing.

—Yeah, but how much does it cost?

"A hundred grand."

Green light.

Jesus fucking Christ!

Chud hasn't started driving yet; he's looking at me.

—That's quite the ticket. I dunno about you, but I don't have that handy. I don't even have half of that handy. I'm pretty heavily invested at the moment, and it'll take a while to sell off. Green.

He looks back to the road and rolls cautiously forward. Unusual. Typically he's a "gas first, check later" sort of guy.

"Yeah. Me too. But think about it, man. It's pure gold. The tag is unreal. Guy just wants rid of it. He's panicking."

—What's the tag per unit?

"Two thousand."

I look out the window and weigh the situation in my mind. This is the big leagues. Is it worth it?

—Good price. But I guess he's desperate. Fifty pounds.

"Fifty kilos …"

We go silent. My muscles tense as if I were about to sprint a hundred metres with a cheetah behind me. My hackles are raised. I'm strapped into the seat, though, and have nowhere

to go. I wish I had access to the gas pedal or the horn. That's
a lot of hash.

—I have an idea.

"I have ears."

* * *

Finding a buyer was the hardest part. We ended up finding a
few separate ones because, realistically, who *really* needs fifty
kilos of Afghani gold-seal hash? Ignoring the fact that it's making a profit off the Taliban, it's also just a ridiculous amount of
hash for one person to buy all in one go. I will, however, point
out that by stealing it we weren't exactly funding the Taliban so
much as just profiting off them. That feels better, I think. We
reached out to Chud's contacts in the local underworld, bikers, my associates from Toronto, and essentially anyone shady
enough to have the buying price on hand in cash. We didn't get
many bites, but the ones we did counted.

We set the price at four thousand a kilo, still a steal by any
stretch or metric, but we stood to make a tidy profit. The issue
remained, though, how to acquire such a gargantuan amount
of the stuff all at once. We just didn't have a hundred thousand
in cash ... or in the bank.

I came by the solution honestly. I was, understandably I'd
say, wary of possibly being pulled over with a duffel bag blooming with federal offences in the trunk, so I wanted to find a
more discreet way to complete the transaction. Chud had a
secret stowaway space in one of his car doors that would accom-
modate about two bricks. I had the idea to do the transaction
over the course of a whole day, in small, safe intervals. Then
it struck me. We'd do the whole transaction that way, money

and hash bit by bit, hand in hand. Instead of picking up fifty kilos and dropping one hundred thousand bucks all at once, we'd only take two kilos at a time, pay four thousand for those, drop them off for eight thousand, and repeat the process every half hour or so, stopping for lunch and smoke breaks. The deal paid for itself by the time it was over, and we each walked away with fifty thousand in profit, from one day of work. The guy only ever had to see us and Juice, who got his finder's cut out of the other guy's proceeds. That was the most I'd ever made in one day.

Over the course of the day, driving from the stash house to the multiple buyers, we passed through a patch of town dominated by strip malls and seedy fast-food joints multiple times. We also happened to pass the police building about fifty times. We nodded at the desk cops having their smokes outside. They waved back at us. Chud knew a few of them. They knew we were good kids.

"Can you imagine working at Tim's? Or McDee's? Man, what, like a hundred bucks a day? Fuck that man. I'd rather do this and risk winding up in prison. At least we're the masters of our own destiny. We punch our own time cards."

—For now.

Chud had a checkered past, to say the least. He'd gone to juvie at seventeen for stealing meat from a grocery store and re-selling it at slashed prices. Just grimy crime. He was no stranger to being down and out.

"Dude, honestly, when the apocalypse comes, it's gonna be me and you just conquering shit. Bahaha, we'll be warlords."

—Huh, I always thought I'd make a good warlord.

"The best. But think about it. We've got all the cash, all the drugs, we can get weapons, we know how to steal, and

we'd fuckin' dominate these civilized people you see going to
work every day if it came down to it. Just wait man. It's gonna
fuckin' happen."

Looking out my window at the homeless kids begging for
sandwiches and heroin money outside of a Quiznos manned by
a teenager with bags under her eyes, all under the bleary gaze of
the cop half passed out in his car in the parking lot, I fiddled
with the growing lump of cash in my pocket and idly wondered
if the apocalypse had already come and gone, more slowly than
any of us had expected or realized. Less of an explosion.

—Let's just keep our heads down and get through it.

THIRTY-TWO

Retrospective:
Bad Influences 2012–2016

I was desperate. Or "desperate." I wasn't, y'know, on death's door, or even just in withdrawal, just pre-eminently bored, frustrated with my situation, and angry at both the world and myself. I'd dutifully waited through my probation period, always in fear of a piss test that never came, and it was finally over. No more visits to the sketchy office. No more condescending social workers. Graduation? Not quite, but I felt like a celebration, with a specific sort of ceremony.

I reached out to one of the wee minions of the Man's little brother. One of the ones who said he could help with anything

I might need. The one of the two who offered their numbers who seemed to be business about it. I'll call him Xerxes.

"Whatchu need man?"

—Whatcha got?

"Weed, coke, crack, oxy, M ... I can get more if you need it."

—I'll go for some coke and oxy. Say, forty bucks of each?

"I got you."

Damn. Good coke. I could tell it was cut with novocaine, but he told me as much before I did it. Jolly decent of him. Here we go again.

I kept my consumption low for a while. I managed functionally. I only had so much money, and it wasn't enough to get properly addicted. I would've been destitute, but once back in the city, Chud made a home call to drop off that care package of twenty thousand dollars and a few grams of DMT. What a sweetheart. I'd been whittling away at that money over a few years, supplementing my income from first a job at a pet store, then a job at a publisher, then as a reconciliation officer at a bank (doing introductory-level accounting). Finally, it ran out just as I was beginning work at The Mercy. Luckily, I'd stumbled across a new form of currency: drug bartering. My access to a multiplicity of high-grade strains and novelty products like shatter, imported hashes, tinctures, Rick Simpson Oil, etc. from Ontario's only semi-legal dispensary far, far, far outpaced the quality of Xerxes's mid-grade street-level shit. Plus I bought ten pounds of high-end mushrooms off my manager at a dirt-cheap hippie price. Cents to the gram type shit. Xerxes didn't have a mushroom link. So the stage was set. He'd give me personal coke, opiates, and MDMA, and I'd keep him in high-grade personal weed and psilocybin.

One day it got complicated. It always does.

—Yo, can I grip an oxy off you today?

"No oxy today, man, sorry."

—What about percs?

There was a long pause.

"I have H."

My turn to pause.

—How much?

"Twenty a point. But fifteen for you today since it's not what you wanted."

—C'mon by, man.

He arrived with a chick he was seeing, a junkie sex worker who'd leave scabs on the floor and needles in the bathroom. She looked beat. She tried singing for us once but stopped short-ly after her voice cracked. I asked if she wanted some water, and she apologized. She started talking to Keeper about Harry Potter. Soon all of us were answering questionnaires to find out what house we belonged to. Apparently I'm a Ravenclaw, and according to the phone, Xerxes was a Slytherin. My girl-friend described what that meant, and he just sort of smiled knowingly.

He had that "I haven't left the dark since I was twelve" look about him, both in the physical and metaphysical senses. He was pale. Tall. Understated. Heavy bags under his eyes, crow's feet, and he'd barely broken twenty. Always wore a nondescript hoodie and baggy jeans, held up at his crack with a faded can-vas belt. He looked like he didn't want to be seen. And I can understand why.

I've never cooked crack. I think. Never sold crack. It was one of Xerxes's favourite activities, though. He'd go on at length about the delicate process and how he'd cut it carefully with a product ironically called "Cutback." He had a dedicated crackhead who'd tell him how hard it hit in exchange for a free rock. And drugs weren't his only game. He'd expanded into other markets. Credit card scams. Malware distribution. Arms dealing. He showed me how he'd legally purchase antique guns online, along with modern parts from separate vendors, then mix and match all the assorted pieces in his possession into functional, untraceable firearms. He'd test them out in the park late at night just to make sure he wasn't selling duds to the sorts of people you don't want to sell defective guns to.

Once we were joking about something, and somehow the situation came up that, if I were walking alone and unarmed and got attacked — like, properly attacked — chased by someone with a gun, or by a whole gang of thugs, of course I'd call the cops to intervene. Especially if I hadn't done anything. This earned a sharp rebuke.

"OK. I'm gonna pretend I never heard that. And if you ever meet my guys, never say anything, ever, about calling the cops. They'll kill you for joking about it."

—Got it.

"Your phone's off, right?"

—Yeah. Of course.

I turn off my phone in my pocket.

"When I'm with my guy, we pull the batteries out and leave them in a different room from where we talk."

This relationship lasted for a few years. I met him in 2012 but couldn't use his drugs for a year, due to probation, so only really knew him from 2013 until about 2016. Long enough to go through quite a bit of money. He kept insinuating himself further into my life. He wanted to start selling his low-grade hash through The Mercy and was putting pressure on me to sell it to my boss. He fronted me a quarter pound as a sampler, but it was garbage. You could barely break into it. Hard as granite and just as smooth on the throat. It was a no go, but he kept pushing me.

This isn't to mention the spiralling nature of my relationship with opioids in this time. I'd gone through percs, oxys, heroin, cold water extract codeine, hydromorphone, promethazine and codeine cough syrup, Dilaudids, etc. I even made poppy seed tea out of desperation when I couldn't contact him. I was deep into it. I never shot up, but I smoked, popped, drank, and snorted anything.

One day I was jonesing hard. I reached out to my trusty Xerxes. He lived a few minutes away, with his dad and sister, and like me, he appreciated punctuality. He'd message me when he was coming, down to the minute — and he'd stick to it.

—Yo, man, I need some down. Carrying?

"Not down, per se. But something similar."

—What is it?

"I'll show you."

Ten minutes later he opened a folded magazine junk packet to display a point of white powder. The heroin he usually brought was slightly brownish, more textured, and sweet smelling. This was just white powder. Could've been flour. Meant nothing to me.

—What is it?

"Fent."

I pause. Adjust to the new reality that I'd already decided to try this powder, no matter what he'd called it.

—How much do I use?

"I cut it down — should be about as strong as the Bayer's H. Start with half, though. Never know. You're the first."

I got the best sleep I'd had in years, from two in the afternoon till four in the morning. Sitting straight up, just nodded
out. Occasionally my eyes opened, fogged like crystal balls,
and I could see the future. I was on a cloud. I was on a river.
I was in the Velvet Underground, sailing darkened seas on a
great big clipper ship, going from this land here to that. I was
home. "Not If You Were the Last Junkie on Earth" was playing
somewhere: something about heroin being cliché. This was no
cliché. This was real. This was new. This was strong.

I messaged Xerxes at five in the morning for more. He was
back at my door in ten minutes. This could be a problem.

One day Xerxes and I were sharing a spliff of some particularly potent Pink Kush. I think he got a little too high, and as
a result, he started talking a bit more than he usually would.
He divulged how some dealers he knew — not him, of course
(according to him) — would sometimes make one batch particularly potent, with the express purpose of not only getting
people higher, but actually *causing* people to OD. Why? When
a junkie hears someone's smack is strong enough to OD from,
at the same price as the usual stuff, they flock to it. Death wish?
No. Simple business. You can use less and get high more often.
They're junkies, not imbeciles. I tried to keep this in mind
going forward and always used half of the intended dose first.
That probably saved me a few times.

I was using fentanyl, and sometimes combining it with coke
as speedballs, for a few months before Xerxes started getting
impatient about the hash deal. He also had his issues with addiction. He was popping Percocets all day, probably using sixty
to eighty milligrams of the active ingredient, oxycodone (the
same opiate in OxyContin), plus all the filler shit they add
to percs. Quantitatively speaking, he was consuming more

opioids than I was. I tried to raise this gently to him one day as he was telling me how tired he was, and he FLIPPED. Do not come between an addict and their addiction unless you're willing to go all the way. He cut me off. No more coke or opes for me. He also demanded his brick of hash back.

Fuck him.

I spent about two hours cutting the brick up into thirds with industrial scissors. I kept one brick, traded another for lower quality coke from another of the Man's little brother's friends, and attached a label to the third: "For Xerxes, in compensation for the good times."

Then I put it in his family's mailbox.

Fuck him.

I saw him around town a few times after this, but we always avoided each other. I knew he regularly carried heat, and he knew I was me. Mutual fear.

Last I heard, he'd been picked up in his early twenties for selling automatic weapons and hefty quantities of narcotics. He's in it for the long haul now.

Fuck him.

THIRTY-THREE

Retrospective on 2016

When I left The Mercy, another guy left, too, hot on my heels. I'll call him Needle. He looked healthy. He looked like Christian Bale. Cut. Slightly noticeable, but still somehow normal nose. Close-set eyes that were always further pushed together by a constant furrowing of his brows. He was always thinking. Always anxious. Needle was also always pissed off at management for not paying us more, or letting us do whatever we wanted at work (which we essentially already did), or any number of other reasons. He had a bone to pick with authority, and in all honesty, he kinda sketched me out. I knew he'd been a reasonably large-scale coke dealer before getting busted and ending up at The Mercy, but there was something more than that — I could tell he had something else wrong either in his

head or hanging over it. Really dedicated to fitness and business. Kind of a Patrick Bateman doppelgänger sort.

Needle still had a few friends in the large-scale herb industry, and he kept bringing samples of their wares to The
Mercy's management, trying to get his finder's fee on the in-
between. We all did it. I had friends from my old 2012 days
who would've loved to get their stuff onto the shelves of The
Mercy, and I tried a number of times, but there was always
someone else willing to drop their prices just a bit more, or who
had an inside relationship with the management and thus got
preferred treatment.

One day while we were both at work, we got to talking.
I didn't really have any interest in doing business with this
guy ... but if money was to be made, I didn't want to be on the
outside of that. I'd been working more and more in the back of
the business, making edibles and extracts. I was the alchemist.
Needle saw potential in this.

"How much do you think they drop on a quarter pound of
shatter here?"

—I haven't made that much at once. For that quantity
they'd buy from outside. But I have no idea. A lot.

"My buddy has a qp. Shatter. Good shit. He wants to sell.
Do you think they'd buy or think they'll just shut it down?"

—Honestly? In my experience, it's a no. They have their
preferred vendors.

"Fuck ... what about if I did something with it? Make
edibles?"

—Same story, man. I make some and they have the Kush
bars from [another employee's connection].

"What about the new dispensaries? Think they'd be looking for stock?"

Now that's an idea.

—Probably not on something like shatter. What you …
what *we* need to do is make something that's not on anyone's
shelves yet.

"Like shrooms or something?"

—No. No, let's try to keep it as legal as possible. Weed
game only. But I've got an idea.

I'd recently begun trying to quit smoking cigarettes. I'd
found gum, the patch, the inhalers, all that shit was garbage.
But I liked the new vaporizers that had only recently become
available, with no medical information available about what
the contents might do to you. They were smooth and discreet,
and they packed a punch the equivalent of raw tobacco. The
only issue was that the liquid was obscenely expensive … so I
bought the components separately. Vegetable glycerin, propylene glycol, and polyethylene glycol 400, along with nicotine
and flavouring. I did my research. I didn't know what the
health implications were, but I knew it was cheaper to make
it myself.

"What's your big idea?"

—Gimme a sec.

I pulled out my phone and started hitting Google hard.
Yup, looked like someone had already done this, and they'd
paved the way with instructions online. I'd have to finagle the
instructions a bit, but I could make it work.

—What about weed vapes? Google says you can make them
with shatter, and I've got the other ingredients already. We'd
just need empty cartridges and a few things to fill them.

"But would they sell? How much would we make?"

—I think if we sold 'em right, they'd sell. And that depends
on how much we can sell them for. The recipe says 0.25 to 0.3

grams of shatter per one millilitre cartridge. But we should make a little batch and hand out samples, see if anyone's even interested before we throw in a qp.

"True, man. True."

Needle was smiling for once.

After a few days I brought a little case of cartridges to work and we gave one to OG, the former junkie and resident cannabis connoisseur, who made the final call on what products we'd carry. He liked it. It was tasty, and even though we told him it was meant as a lighter option than joints, he still felt it a bit.

"What strain is this?"

—Peach Pie.

"This is delicious, guys. But we're not gonna buy it. I don't know enough about what's inside."

That's pretty much the response I'd expected. Needle was pissed. After work we got on the streetcar along Queen West and stopped at every dispensary, giving a cartridge and battery to the manager of each spot we passed through. It was time to spread our wings and branch out from The Mercy. We got a number of hits. A few locations decided to tentatively buy ten or so cartridges at a time. Not exactly big numbers, but they would hopefully add up. We got to work that weekend turning shatter into e-juice and stacking cartridges.

My recipe was straightforward and mostly stolen. I'd mix 0.3 grams of shatter with 0.55 millilitres of propylene glycol and 0.15 millilitres of polyethylene glycol 400 to emulsify it properly, then microwave that in a glass vial for thirteen seconds, stir, and transfer from the vial to the cartridge using a syringe. Each cartridge cost us about four dollars to make, then we'd sell them at twenty-five dollars apiece in allotments of ten, twenty dollars apiece in allotments of fifty, and fifteen dollars apiece in allotments of one hundred. Negotiable above one hundred. We worked out the details of how the business would operate at my kitchen table, each of us speed-filling cartridges, the microwave pinging every few seconds.

—You want anything to eat?

"Oh shit, my meds. No, it's OK. I brought my own food, but I need to take my meds."

—Oh yeah … you're really health conscious, eh?

"Well, I have to be."

—Like, more so than the average human?

"Do you not know?"

—Know what?

"I have HIV, man."

Oh shit …

—Oh shit … sorry, man.

"It's fine, dude. I got it the worst way. I'd never done anything intravenous, but I was doing a lot of meth and snorting and smoking, and it wasn't getting me where I needed to be, so my buddy gave me his needle. He had HIV, though, and I got it. Haven't used meth or coke or a needle since. It, like, freaked me out. I work really hard to stay healthy. Like, I'm twenty-five. I don't wanna die yet."

Makes sense. Me neither.

Business was good. Our people had gone through their initial sales and received positive feedback, so they upped their orders. We were getting multiple orders above one hundred cartridges. This felt almost like the old days, just more wholesome. We even started supplying a few dispensaries with kaya from either my own or Needle's amigos from the old days, but most places could beat our prices with their connections out west.

Then the cops came. Not for us, but for the dispensaries. We'd go to make a drop and see boards over the doors: redundant what with most of them being made of reinforced steel, with bars protecting the windows pre-closure, but the government needed to make a statement, I guess. They came with SWAT teams to freak the shit out of the barely out of high school–aged cashiers and strike the fear of "Legislation" into them. They came with battering rams during rush hour. It was a publicity stunt. A ploy to clear the streets of the old guard in anticipation of legalization: something the higher-ups had a personal stake in. I tip my cap to the former Hash King of Etobicoke. You played your hand well.

Going legit was the highest prize of all — and something worth causing some shit over.

It was good while it lasted, but in no time at all our entire business evaporated. Memories of a dream fading into a stressful day. We were stuck with about a hundred cartridges, a few pounds of weed, and a quarter pound each of Peach Pie and Lemon Haze shatter. It was all at my place. I told Needle we should lay low for a while before emerging and offering our services again to the new generation of dispensaries replacing the old guard. He agreed, and we went radio silent.

I haven't heard from Needle since. I smoked or sold all the stuff, so I kinda hope I don't hear from him … but I do hope he's OK. One sketchbag to another.

THIRTY-FOUR

2002 Onward: Retrospective on Business Chat

So, you know about my first time getting high, when I watched Dark Side of Oz. How did that transition into the life I've led, though? Well, it's a fairly straightforward story, really.

Three and a half grams of weed, that's what you call a half-quarter (of an ounce … Americans call them "eighths") or an "hq." That's pretty much the standard purchasing increment for most people at the recreational scale. Sure, occasionally you get someone looking for the bulk deals beyond an ounce, or some trepidatious or poverty-stricken kid looking for only one gram, but by and large, half-quads are meant for consumption.

I didn't know that, though. At least not at twelve. The first
day I got back to school, I bought three and a half grams with
the express intent of getting that half gram for free. I'd paid
thirty bucks for some electric-green leafy buds covered in red
hairs and what looked like a dusting of granular sugar. This is
the weed that I would one day know as M-39. Low THC, easy
to grow, headache stone … we knew it as "Asian" because it
was allegedly coming from East Asian gangs across southern
Ontario, but it was just as likely an epithet garnered by either
a well-intentioned comparison to old-school Thai Stick weed
or out-and-out racism. Anyway, I managed to convince three
other kids to buy a gram apiece (and silly me not having a scale,
eyeing it out with a tendency toward conservatism). Let's just
say the half gram left over looked pretty fat.

And that was it. I was a dealer. I could blaze for free. No
looking back now.

Pretty soon I was immersed in the world of entry-level dealing. It was fun. There was a culture. There were challenges
requiring creativity and a few heart-thumping seconds of luck
to not get caught. Hiding Baggies in interesting places, like the
snow pile next to the soccer field, or in the middle of a PB&J
sandwich. Escaping the watchful eyes of parents and teachers,
and even police; it was a game, and I won every time.

I spent high school getting more acquainted with the in-
tricacies of the drug game and sampling more products, but I
never bought in huge amounts. An ounce at most, in general,
and always just to fuel my own consumption. That's the mindset I left for university with.

I arrived in my dorm room in 2007 with an ounce to win
over my new dorm mates. In a charming display of happenstance, my roommate (Teddy) showed up with a quarter

pound. We decided to form a team and smoke the profits equally.

Once we ran out of our initial supply, we obviously needed to re-up. Problem was, we were at school, and nobody was willing to drive an order between an ounce and a quarter pound from our respective cities. There just wasn't enough profit in it to justify the gas and risk of highway patrol. Out of desperation, we resorted to buying off a scuzzbag. I'll call him Frat Boy.

Frat Boy was a pasty kid, always sporting some variety of blended professional basketball or baseball or football or hockey paraphernalia from a different city every few days, often during the wrong season: Celtics jersey with a Bruins hat in June sort of thing. He lived in our building but on a different floor. A stagnant five-o'clock-shadow creep who'd take pictures of his bowel movements and send them to our dormitory group chats, tagging the girls he liked that week. "Guys, you gotta try working out. Chicks love it and it makes your dick bigger." Last thing he needed was to be a bigger dick.

I didn't like Frat Boy for a number of reasons, but the one that really got me pissed was his prices. Two hundred bucks an ounce for moist, black-ash-burning shite. The worst part was how he justified it: "Guys, I have to charge that much. I'm Jewish." No, dude. Own your own shitty disposition; don't cop out as an intentional stereotype.

We bought off Frat Boy a few times. More than we'd wanted to, but we were simultaneously laying the foundations for a plan that would disrupt his operations, and we wanted to do it right.

Somehow we'd been introduced (by our, for lack of a better word, "friend" with a coke habit) to another local dealer … a little larger in scale, and a little more diverse in what he carried.

Juice. Juice was fit. That was his thing. He actually played the sports Frat Boy made childish long-shot bets on. He kept a personal grooming schedule worthy of a designer bar of soap. Guy was sharp-lookin'. He was a consummate professional. He was smart. He was someone who could teach us things.

Juice was also Jewish (and no, that's not why he's called "Juice") and countered Frat Boy's self-centred anti-Semitism with great prices on drugs. His low-grade weed was one hundred and sixty for an ounce, but it looked a helluva lot better than Frat Boy's shitty outdoor AK-47. At least Juice's stuff was indoor hydro. We bought an ounce and brought it back with a plan. We were going to charge thirty dollars for a half-quarter, the way it should be, the way we'd all come to expect it until Frat Boy decided to charge forty for a half-quarter. But we weren't doing it to smoke for free. We were going to sell that ounce for two hundred and forty dollars (we'd advertised to all of Frat Boy's customers we knew) and then we were going to add that eighty-dollar earnings to what we could buy, and just sort of go from there. The half-quarters would cost the same for all of us, Teddy and I included: thirty dollars. We'd have to pay in the same way everyone else did. I figured that would keep consumption low and stop us from bickering over who smoked which nug, etc.

I went back to Juice's place three more times that day, eventually carrying four hundred bucks over the threshold in the hopes of buying that fourth ounce when he said something along the lines of:

"Listen, bro, you're nice and everything, but I can't have you coming by four times a day. It looks sketch."

—Fair enough ... but what else then? I can't grab more than a couple zips at a time yet ... but I've got mad demand.

"K. How 'bout I take this four hundo as a down payment and front you ... maybe, hmm ... a pound? You think you could move that in a week or so? I'll tag that at fifteen bills, for now, minus this four hundo."

—Man, I can't promise anything for sure. That's a lot of weed.

"Just take it and see where you go."

Something told me Juice had a lot more of this stuff sitting in his cupboards ... I was being groomed for something.

I was back within a day or two, sold right out. I'd even made enough (on top of that initial down payment) to outright buy my own weed; I didn't need the loan anymore. I got some bonus pissed-off voice mails from Frat Boy threatening me and Teddy if we didn't stop taking his business. I decided to go for broke and dropped the price on the half-quarter to twenty-five. I had more calls coming through my phone than I had time to fill the Baggies for their orders.

We started expanding the selection of varietals we carried. We got into lows, mediums, highs. Hashes. The odd honey oil. Mushies. We'd always carry a few different strains: it's just good business. Never build a company around one product. I'd learned things from sitting at the table with my parents while we discussed geopolitics and global commerce over dinner ... something I intend to do if and when I have my own family. Maybe my kids will grow up to slang product, too. If they do, they'd better do it proper.

In next to no time we put Frat Boy flat out of work, and business with Juice was booming. We'd gotten to a point where we'd not only taken most of his customers, but I'd found out who his supplier was. I already knew their weed was garbage from when I'd been forced to buy off that shithead Frat Boy in the first place, so I knew they had at least one weak spot.

—I can beat what you're getting. You're getting low-grade shit, and I can guess what you pay for it, and I think you're overpaying. Let me help you.

The dealer wasn't any sort of business person. He was just a kid in a higher position than was deserved. But he wasn't stupid.

"Yeah? What's your offer?"

—A grand for a half nut. Eighteen hundred for the full thing.

I'd estimated that he was likely paying more like seven, seven-fifty on a quarter pound. Twelve to thirteen for a half. So on the face of it my offer was superior, but he kept his cool. Money was one thing; the product itself was another.

I pulled a full half-pound vacuum-sealed bag out of my knapsack. The right way to show merchandise.

—This is what it looks like.

I wanted to make sure he had the full experience. Nothing quite compares to opening up one of those bags and sticking your whole face in for a taste of the terps, aside from visiting the actual production facilities. I pulled out my knife and cut the top of the bag off and handed it to him. Juicy Fruit. His face lit up like a kid picking the Christmas tree.

"I think we good."

—Cool. One last request: don't fuck with [Frat Boy] anymore. We want him out.

I was expecting some sort of "But, he's my boy!" or "I can't turn down that much business" response. But my offer must have really exceeded his expectations.

"Done, broski. This shit is insane. Smells like a fucking grapefruit covered in rat piss … in, like, the best possible way."

Frat Boy was still around, selling my weed as grams to friends and the desperate, but his moment in the sun had passed. Dumbass wasn't even nineteen yet, and he'd peaked.

It was shortly after this point in time that I had a falling out with Teddy. I was, well, not necessarily "well" through all of this. I was dealing with some strange feelings I'd had my whole life, which were getting substantially more overwhelming as I adapted to living away from home, conducting my schooling (here and there), running a growing business, and self-medicating for a disorder I didn't yet know I had.

I came to believe Teddy was stealing from me. There was so much money flowing through our business that it was inevitable some would get lost, but the sickness inside told me it was someone else's fault. And, nobody could argue, Teddy was sloppy: even if he was losing money by accident, that was still a lot of money. So I broke the business in half. I took half the money, I took Juice, and I took my leave. I moved out and set up in a pixie pad. A new home from which to profit and proselytize about the benefits of the dankest peng available.

I'm not the best by myself, though — what, after all, is a Mad Hatter without a March Hare? I had to restructure my organization accordingly: enter Chud. We met in a class on ancient Western philosophy. I liked Diogenes, he liked Marcus Aurelius. We bonded. It didn't take long for the conversation to come around to weed. And the weed talk didn't last long before we started talking business.

It had always been fun, dodging cops, making money, getting drugs for free. But chopping with Chud took it to another level. We'd become kingpins.

I'd started selling pot all those years ago as a way to feed my habit — and that had been the general rule for most of my adolescence — but once you start making more money than you can smoke up, well, that's an addiction in itself. It feels like Monopoly money, it comes and goes so quickly. Charge your buddy a thousand for something you charge a stranger two thousand for. The prices can be so arbitrary, but they follow certain rules. How well do I know you? Do I like you? Do I know you have other options in the drug-purchasing experience, or are you stuck with me? How much is my competition charging you? Fuck, even, is rent due this week and can I squeeze this chump for a few grand? The rubber-band rolled bundles of five thousand filled up our safes in no time, and we had to get rid of it somehow. We were too addicted to the game to retire cold turkey. Buy the whole bar dinner, drinks, and dessert? Why not? I don't have another pocket to stuff anyway.

I drunkenly lost clothing and backpacks with more than the annual Canadian average wage several times. I'd misplace ten thousand like a pair of keys. Oops. Guess it's time to make another flip. Hope I made a hobo happy.

Heart palpitations are fucked. But they sure do make you appreciate life. Dodging the sound of the whoop-whoop has a similar effect. It's like free climbing. One wrong leap and you're either sharing a cell with some scary-ass fucker or getting shot in the back by a service pistol. And while your average citizen might intuitively avoid such circumstances, Chud and I sought them out.

Not only all that, but you have to remember that we were consuming several hundred dollars' worth of assorted substances a day. We needed to keep that lifeline for our personal stash open. And the best way to do that is to buy in bulk. We were addicted to all of it. Even all my friends were somehow involved, either as lieutenants or indirectly somehow through drug culture — graffiti, music, skateboarding, street kids, and anarchists, etc. I spent a lot of time chilling with my street friends at a local shelter. I scrawled poetry on the walls. I handed out weed and mushrooms for free: my version of charity. We jammed. I'd play guitar or sing my songs, and then we'd collapse in drug comas, careful to avoid the discarded needles and bathroom from whence constant plumes of plastic-smelling crack-smoke clouds were coming.

It was impossible to escape unless you were just sort of scooped out and isolated, deprived of the drugs and the friends and the excitement. And I guess that's sort of what happened to me. For the best, in retrospect.

After all that, though, the years spent in a black-market industry, the vast sums of knowledge about biochemistry, toxicology, microeconomics, marketing, scaring the shit out of punk-ass muthafuckas, comes the real-life job search. It's hard. It's more than switching careers, it's explaining why you're more than qualified for a role while skirting around huge blank periods on your resumé. Especially now you're just sort of meant to shoot your CV into the black hole of the email realm. LinkedIn is for chumps. And I have to be one of them. If you can, though … nepotism is where it's at.

THIRTY-FIVE

Retrospective on 2015

After spending more than a while at the computer, each application gnawing off another part of my soul, my dad must've taken some pity on me. He put out feelers to see if anyone at the bank could find an entry-level position for me — something that would make use of my keen eye for details and keep me away from the more nuanced aspects of high finance that I had yet to learn.

With some degree of luck, I was landed a position as a reconciliation officer (and I still can't quite explain what that is …). I say "I was landed" instead of "I landed" because my dad's buddy sat in on my interview and basically intimated something along the lines of "Hire this kid or it's your ass." He looked like George Costanza living off a diet of success, who had come to expect things to go his way. I'd made an absolute fool of myself in the interview, but I got hired in Capital Markets. They said it was the most cutthroat department of the bank. Gulp.

After a few days of training I took nothing from, I was released onto the stage of international finance. Before we even get into the job itself, let me say that I'd never had an office job. I only knew what to expect through popular media's depictions of what was going on. Figuring out the coffee machine took a while. And I never figured out where the extra folders and pens and shit were kept ... I'd just steal them from other people after it became embarrassingly late to ask someone.

The first two weeks were normal nine-to-five type days, but I knew the schedule would be variable. There was, well, a lot to take in. Daily grooming for me is tough. There's a pragmatic reason I rock a beard now. Then I couldn't. I had to be the clean-cut company man. This was next level. This was, like, computers and stuff. Whoa.

I put a plant and some of my dark little cartoons in my cubicle. People were superficially friendly. Some might have actually been friendly, but they blended in so well with the predominant personality type: predator. I was spoken to when I spoke to people. So that how it be, eh?

My job, I think, was to match portions of trades with each other. I would see that someone had sold however much of one thing and someone else had bought the same amount of the same thing, so then I'd tie them together ... easy, right? Sometimes, though, you had one trade coming in as separate parts, and the parts I was trying to match them to would be different but add up to the same. Then again, sometimes a chunk of the trade was missing, or the same item at the same value was traded by multiple actors in one session, so I'd have to trace specific blocks of trade.

To try to trace this mind-jumbling array of decimal points and currency symbols, I used anywhere from five to ten pieces of software, which all changed regularly, all with different passwords that also changed every few days, and it made no sense whatsoever. What did I expect? I never studied any of this shit. I could barely track my drug inventory in Excel. Add to this the fact that my shifts began to swing all around the clock. So I would regularly be the only person on my floor at 3:00 a.m. trying to make this fucking time-sensitive puzzle work — well, the only person apart from the Portuguese cleaner who probably had greater insight to the finer details of the market than I did. Anyway, inevitably as I was closing up my computer, I'd start getting angry calls from Hong Kong, Sydney, or Singapore, from actual financiers pissed to the tits at my sweeping up of their previous day's trades.

One night at about three or four in the morning, I had a moment of crisis. I hit a breaking point. I was supposed to be done in about an hour, and I'd thought I was going to be done early, even able to skip out home for the last hour, with none the wiser, nobody watching me as long as the work was done. But I ran into an issue. I'd tied together about a thousand or so trades and was getting to the end. This was the easiest bit. Like putting in the last few jigsaw pieces. Then, fuck … there was one trade left. It was worth a few cents. A vestigial financial organ. Like an appendix set to burst in my face in an hour. But I couldn't close the system without having found its match (which I must've matched by accident some time ago, into some other trade). So basically, I was searching for where a few cents fit into a spreadsheet carrying upward of a hundred billion dollars ... fuck, a needle in a haystack. I wished I could just use a magnet on the computer monitor.

I started freaking out. I emailed the people who needed to know, but they were either asleep or on their way to work already, assuming I had my end in order. I had no idea what to do. I couldn't go back and uncouple all those trades; I'd never have the time. And while I knew that people got pissed over this, I didn't really understand how these few missing cents would impact the global market.

WHY WAS I NOT TRAINED FOR THIS?!

I lost it, so I called my dad. What did he know about reconciliations? Probably not much more than me, but I wasn't thinking clearly. He actually woke up, got dressed, and drove the half hour to my office building on King Street to help me troubleshoot. I had about fifteen minutes left by the time he got there before I was expecting some pissed-off Aussie stockbroker accents screaming down my phone line. My dad was fairly nonchalant. He seemed more concerned about me than the few cents that might break the market's back.

"So, what do we do?"

Motherfucker's wearing a suit. He looks like Pierce Brosnan about to do some epic shit. He kitted out, cuffs and all, just to walk through the building. My sleeves are rolled up, my tie is loosened, my shirt is untucked, and my back is soaked with sweat.

—I don't fuckin' know! That's why I called you! I'm freaking out!

"Well, did you tell the people who need to know?"

—Yeah.

"Then there's not much more you can do."

What?

—But the market …

"There's nothing you can do. They didn't teach you how to do your job. That's on them. Want my advice?"

—Yeah, Dad.

"Let's go home. Get you to bed."

—But they're gonna start calling soon!

"And they'll get your voice mail. And if they're really pissed, they can call me."

There are benefits to power. And privileges in proximity to power. And power has its prerogatives.

Bed did sound nice …

Know what? Fuck 'em. I worked for that bank for six miserable months and figured that was enough to start my resumé up again. I turned down the three-month contract extension they'd offered (probably on the threat of dead-end careers if they hadn't) and finished my last few days in a flurry of I-don't-give-a-fucks. They must've had someone behind the scenes doing all the work I wasn't doing … or maybe my work had just never been that vital all along. I don't know and don't care. It's behind me. I quit.

THIRTY-SIX

August 13, 2017, 1:53 a.m.

I have this friend from high school — let's call him Big Poppa Smurf, or Smurf, for short — whom I hadn't spoken to for three years (for reasons relating to lots of drugs and my instability, as usual). He'd always been one of my more stable buddies — studied engineering and always had a job and a girlfriend. Shit-together sorta person. Well anyway, he texted me from the waiting room of the CAMH emergency ward. And as it turned out over the last three years, he's bipolar as fuck as well. It just didn't really kick in until his midtwenties. Takes all types to make a world.

So Smurf was asking me questions and explaining his situation by text, then I got a text from another old buddy I hadn't heard from for years, and he was saying he'd just dropped

Smurf off at the hospital and Smurf was really insistent on talking to me (thinking I was the only person who would get what he was saying) … I understood the feeling; when you're manic or psychotic, you instinctively don't trust doctors, but really, there's only so much I can do by text, with someone who's super-manic, and whom I haven't spoken to since before he got, like, *clinically* sick. I just kept it super simple: encouragement, validation, advice on what meds I've found most useful in those situations, and generally just stuff like, "It's best to do what the doctors say. They're not actually evil." Oh, he also spent last night in jail … so there's a legal component to all of this, which means you *really* have to follow the doctor's orders. I'm keeping my eyes on the situation, but there's not much more I can do, so I start watching *Fantasia*. That 1940s steez. Not this millennium shit. I'm getting ready for bed.

About half an hour after the last texts back and forth, by which time I assumed he was being seen in the well-secured admission room, I was rolling a doobie for a stroll when I got a text from the second buddy:

"[Smurf] just pulled a runner on CAMH. He said he was going out for a smoke and he disappeared."

Fuck.

He's skipping out on bail. Right off the bat, that's a life-fucking move. Plus he doesn't have any meds — not that he'd probably be taking them, but at least if he had some benzos, he could get some sleep and control his agitation. Instead he has weed, cigarettes, and readily available alcohol all over the place, plus whatever else you can find on the streets of downtown Toronto while manic (which is pretty much anything). I finish up spinning a spliff. I lick the glue, fold the paper over, pack the bouquet down with a chopstick, find my shoes, and get outside, where I have a perambulatory pattern planned out. I start off in stride.

My phone starts ringing a few minutes after that message. Unidentified number. Fuck's sake.

—Hey, man.

"Hey! How's it going? Long time no see, eh? Or talk. Ha-ha-ha! What's up with you? How's life been? Oh, it's [Smurf] by the way. Yeah, I know. Sorry about the last few years, man. I feel really bad. Like, really *really* bad. I don't know what happened. But, yeah, I'm, like, I'm, uhh ... I'm sorry! And, well, anyway, I'm having, like, some issues, or whatever. Wait! You already know, right?. I was just talking to you? Yeah!"

—Yeah, man. We were just talking to each other, remember? It's me, man. Don't worry about what happened. We've both been through some tough times. I just wanna know — where are you?

"Ha-ha-ha-ha! Good try, buddy! Nicely played, buddy-boy! Well done! But you're gonna have to do better than that if you're working for *them*. I'm not a mouse, *duuude*! I don't do tricks and surrender for cheese."

—Look, I know what the inside of your head feels like right now. I'll tell you that I'm not trying to get you. But you feel like you can't trust anyone — not even yourself — from moment to moment, right? All I'm trying to do is what's best for you.

"Ha-ha-ha! Don't fuckin' do that, *man*! Ha-ha-ha-ha. Like, don't even try, buddy. You think you're the shit and you're *sooo* fuckin' smart and you can just do anything, but I'm, like, I'm on, like, beyond the world of levels. I'm not even in your fuckin' *world*, man!"

—You called me, remember? Right? You called me for *help*: because you know that I can do *that*. So where are you? Where are you going?

"I'm in an Uber headed to an unknown location."

—Like, an *undisclosed* location? Or unknown?

"Both! Then, I dunno, maybe I'll go to BC. Or maybe I'll lay low for a little while then go to my court date. That'll look good, right? Like, good behaviour and everything?"

—Dude, you skipped bail. There is no court date. The best, best, *best* thing you can do right now is go back to CAMH. I can't force your hand, but I can say, one fuckup to another, that's your best course of action.

"What … What if I lay low for, like, two weeks, and I come back and I'm not fucked up anymore, and I go to CAMH then?"

—I dunno, man. I'm not a lawyer. It … I guess it could work, but —

"OK! Thanks, buddy! You're a lifesaver!"

He hangs up. Fuck's sake. Why does everybody always call me?

I flick the remaining half of the joint. I don't feel like getting that high anymore. It flies straight down a storm drain. At least something's going right tonight. I head home and resume *Fantasia*'s Tchaikovsky mushroom-dance lullaby sequence.

THIRTY-SEVEN

August 13, 2017, 5:14 p.m.

Today has a theme. Maybe there's just a proliferation of madness around me, on the other hand. I do seem to attract a strange sort ... always have. And it never rains but pours. If I were really, truly insane, I'd say it had something to do with astrology.

I was at the top of my parents' street a few hours ago, on the way to Bloor, and ran into my childhood neighbour buddy — we'll call him Pole (on account of his lankiness ... there is absolutely no ethnic/nationalistic connotation to his name — just wanna be clear).

Now, I'd heard through the gossip-vine that he'd had some issues of his own over the winter. Something about him pacing while naked (outside) in February and being trucked off to emergency by armed people. He was kneeling down and sorting through a few leaves, pebbles, and chunks of dirt — for what, I haven't the foggiest. I slowed down awkwardly ...

—Yo, wassup?

"Good. You?"

He'd never been strong, conversationally. But he was always a nice guy. Probably one of my best friends from childhood. His parents ran a deli, and I remember one day his mom coming back with chocolate for us: "Is Polish chocolate. Number two chocolate in world." I guess he came by his conversational skills honestly. His mom sounds like a Bram Stoker version of Princess Diana. Very pleasant lady, but when she asks you if you want a sandwich, it feels like you don't have a choice. He learned English at her feet.

I try to meet his gaze:

—Good, man. And not much.

"Oh, yeah."

—So ... wassup?

"Oh, yeah ... huh-huh."

—Uhh ... yeah.

I guess I have to think of him differently now. I remember spending endless hours playing N64 with him. Chilling out to Zelda puzzles and racing in *Mario Kart*. Then *Grand Theft Auto* on PlayStation, going on murder sprees and fantasizing about being gangsters someday. He was one of the first two kids I got high with.

—I heard you had a tough winter. How's that going? I've been there, man. No judgment. Didn't know if you knew.

"Oh, yeah ... huh-huh."

I decided to see if he'd forward any more information if I didn't pursue.

"Yeah. I got, like, sick. Like, mental shit. Yeah. Huh-huh."

—How do you feel now?

"I don't think I should be here yet. Huh."

We hadn't made eye contact yet.

—Do you need anything? Like, I can talk with you or tell you about programs or whatever.

"Yeah. Huh-huh."

—OK. Well, I'm on my way to the gym now. The place you used to go. If you wanna start again, we could always go together.

"Yeah. Huh-huh."

—Yeah. And, if you need anything then just give me a holler, eh? Just knock on the door. You're not alone.

"Yeah."

—Easy out, man.

"Easy out. Yeah."

THIRTY-EIGHT
September 12, 2017

I've met a new girl. More than a friend, but not a girlfriend. And more than "just" a girl, or so it seems right now. I've tentatively given her the rough manuscript of this book, which she's reading now. She's also a writer in her own right, so it's not totally insane — or so I'm saying.

We met online. The sensible way, to me, at least. Where you can screen out most of the crazy. Strange as it may sound to some, online dating is less about appearance and more of a personality filtering mechanism, at least to me. Chuckles only had one picture: a bad one, if I may say. Her photo didn't give me much to work off, but her profile seemed at least interesting. She had a sense of humour and thoughts.

The platform would give you a personality quiz, trying to match you up with potential mates who'd responded accordingly, but you could really get into the answers in the comment section. She was making obscure Trump jokes deep in the nether-realm of dating. There were lists of her favourite TV shows, books, movies, and music. We synced up with regularity. Saying she was vibing off *Rick and Morty* was a foregone conclusion. She obviously hadn't put much serious thought into her self-synopsis, saying she was studying literature at the University of Toronto and littering the page with typos and grammatical bellyflops. She said she was only looking for friends, but I sent her a message:

—Hi. You seem a fair bit like me. If you like yourself, then maybe you'll like me too.

She responded soon after:

"Hi, me."

Our messages continued. The topic strayed to substance use, as it so often does with me, but also for transparency:

—I smoke pot now every couple days, but that's pretty much it. I used to do everything, though, and in extreme volumes.

"By 'do everything,' I'm going to think ... everything. That's madness. Well done on being able to stop. I assume that was near impossible. But you're basically Pickle Rick, so I'd expect no less."

—Because you called me Pickle Rick, you get my phone number.

On my phone her contact title is "Chuckles Skullfucker," which was the culmination of a nicknaming duel we had today. Her name for me is the Rickdiculous. We'd met right after the "Pickle Rick" episode came out ... she says that Jerry is the most relatable character.

She sees me as a near otherworldly fey-land creature, half magic, half science, all absurdity — herself coming from a fairly conservative family and growing up fairly sheltered and me being all like, "I used to take industrial doses of acid on the regular."

I feel confident that she is a phenomenal woman. It's early days … just shy of a month. But she seems pretty cool so far. And I can be a good judge of character. She hits all the check marks of the getting-to-know-you protocol. Plus she's kinda weird. She questions things … definitely. And not in the ways I would. And she's brave — but also terrified of the world at large. She's a lot like me in the sense that she seems like a centenarian/six-year-old in the same sentence. Great sense of humour. She's had an interesting past, which she can say more about in her own words.

I invited her to a literary event as my date … probably a bit awkward for her, though, since she was a stranger and most of the attendees were friends and acquaintances of mine. My bad. I'm not good at wooing. When we finally met in person, we were both nervous, but she was visibly shaking. We met at a restaurant patio on Spadina, within view of the College Street CAMH location I'd been held in last year. This was before the event: an early September shindig held in the parking lot behind a small but notable publishing house. An industry incest fest.

She'd never done the whole "online thing" before, and it was a bit much to meet a strange man (who'd told her all these stories, by the way). She asked if we could just sit in silence for about five minutes. Just to calm her nerves.

—Sure.

Silence. I looked at my phone. It went on for eight or so minutes. She's not good at time.

Fuck. She's beautiful. I had no idea this was coming. That was a really bad picture on her profile. She really gave absolutely no fucks about that site. This date is providence. She had mentioned she's not photogenic. I thought that was intended to prepare me for something she thought would disappoint me. She's a sprite, though. A tiny little thing just full of child-like wonder and mischief. She has a timeless look. Like she's a Tolkien character with a Cymraeg-based name. She's Noldor. Older than she looks and younger than she seems. She must be made of magic. That or I just scored that classic cliché of a hat trick: smart, funny, and beautiful. I thought I wasn't one of those guys with a type, but she's mine.

—You OK?

She seemed spaced the fuck out.

"Sorry, sometimes I dissociate when I'm really anxious."

—Take your time. Should I order a pitcher?

She was quick to respond.

"Yes! Please, I mean. I mean … I like beer. I'm kind of freaking out. Beep-boop. Daria words …"

—I couldn't tell.

She made eye contact, gave me a cockeyed look, and smiled: "Fuck you."

—Would that I were so lucky.

"Just for friends!"

—Why are you so anxious then?

"The event."

I waited for her to make eye contact again. It took about thirty seconds of silence.

—Sure.

The beer arrived and she ordered chicken nuggets. The fuck?

—Nugs?

"Shut up! They're comfort food!"

We danced around the flirting like a flitting fly around a light. We drank beer. Another pitcher. I ate a nug in solidarity. Then I ate another.

"Fuck off. Them's my nugs."

She had a touch of a glow in her cheeks.

—I paid for them.

She pursed her lips.

"As friends."

—Sure.

Then we walked to the party. It was poppin', and she was jaw-droppin' at the company we were keeping. She met the Godfather. He was excited to see me for the first time since this same party the year before.

"Yo, man! Wanna smoke some weed?"

I still didn't know how Chuckles felt about casual consumption of drugs. I knew she wasn't opposed to my smoking pot occasionally, but how often did *occasionally* connote? She was sitting on some steps toward the back of the parking lot, listening to our conversation with a deeply furrowed brow, surveying the Godfather.

—I'm good, man.

He leaned in closer:

"How about some coke?"

He leaned back and smiled the smile of a sacred secret holder, almost like everyone in the circle hadn't heard him. They all looked at me:

—Again, gonna hold off on that.

"Fair enough, man. Well, I'm gonna go talk to people."

—OK.

He paused. Possibly remembering about the existence of societal norms. Right, you're supposed to talk to people you haven't seen in a year, even if they aren't getting fucked up with you.

"Are you working on anything right now?"

—I mean, I've got a bunch of poems. And I started doing some comics lately. I'd love to land a publisher for those. I'm also working on, like, a creative non-fiction memoir type thing. Are you working on anything?

"Yeah, man! I've got a chapbook coming out soon, and I've got a few deals in the making with a couple of places for a few other things. I'm writing a lot."

—That's great, man.

I guess he wasn't interested in my projects. It's OK; I guess I wasn't that interested in his. Once he'd walked away, Chuckles turned to me, a free sausage undergoing mastication as she opened her mouth and tumbled:

"Interesting friend."

—Yeah, he's got basically the same diagnosis as me.

"Interesting."

The rest of the night passed like a fairy tale. I found some random unfortunate editor and uninvitedly began reciting spoken word at her with no purpose whatsoever and to no applause. I was getting a bit sloppy off the freely traded drink tickets. Chuckles found the only other person at the party who played Dungeons & Dragons, and they chatted it up for about half an hour. I took Chuckles on a whirlwind tour of the rickety old publishing house. I showed her the ancient printing machine, the drafty bathroom (from which she stole a sci-fi magazine from the fifties, further bolstering my view of her), and the upstairs library, complete with a very old chair that, according to legend, has been subjected to the farts of many of Canada's greatest literary minds. I sat on the chair and farted my mark. She sat on me ... she didn't leave a mark, but I felt it, regardless.

At the end of the night we retired to a parkette and sat on a bench. She put her head on my shoulder and looked up. I made eye contact:

—Just friends?

She smiled and blushed and squished her face into my chest and made a muffled "*fuck*" sound, then spun around and looked at me very seriously:

"This might be a problem."

It worked, though. We're still talking. And it's fantastic so far.

THIRTY-NINE
December 22, 2017

When bumming a smoke on the street, a few simple tactics will significantly increase your odds of success, but they vary in application according to circumstance.

Offering remuneration always helps. Different amounts for different targets. Profile them. I find fifty cents to be the most broadly effective. Two quarters, for simplicity. Most people, especially the well-dressed and, for some reason, construction/maintenance workers, will tell you not to worry about it and just give you a cigarette for free … maybe fifty cents is too much hassle to put in your pocket without a high enough pay-out. Occasionally, a loonie is warranted; I usually find this to be when approaching a group outside a bar … say, "'Scuse me, any chance I could buy a smoke off someone?" Then flash the loonie prominently with a smile, almost as though you expect what you're asking for. One of them will rush to show their charitable side and offer the smoke free of charge. It's usually the person with the most expensive brand.

Be well-dressed and clean-cut. Look approachable. You don't want to look like you're begging; you're just between packs. Always smile. Walk as you scan, like a landlubber shark: never stop and loiter … it seems desperate.

For me, at least, young people are the easiest prey. They get it. They've been there recently. We silly millennials, never planning ahead for anything, share comradery and philanthropy like the clap.

After that it's middle-aged women (for me, at least) who'd just never quit and are generally congenial, as long as you're OK with a lingering look and maybe a lasting pat on the arm.

The group with the lowest score, and my demographic of last resort, are middle-aged Caucasian men. They don't even acknowledge me half the time. They speed up and swerve away like you are a sexual-assault allegation. Homeless people are more likely to give you a smoke than baby boomers with new, business-focused branding — but the former take the fifty cents, and their cigarettes are fucking wretched.

When you're selling drugs, similar skill sets are employed, but different tactics.

"Not much left of this one. Everybody's been about it. Just got in and almost out." Putting the pressure of time on someone is often your most powerful tool. Their heart begins racing. Adrenalin pumps. Long-term thinking is delayed, and they focus on the now. Their propensity to take risks increases. They become victims of biology, especially since you're selling a dream. Often, it's one they're addicted to.

Be friendly, but experienced … worldly, and in absolute control. You know the baser side of the world; you've dwelled underground and seen darkness; you have a thousand light year stare; but your customers are too small fry to elicit your wrath. All they have to do is wipe their shoes at the door, kowtow, buy their drugs in deference, and pay — they'll be safe. Be a good and bad cop in one fell swoop.

Always keep a variety of products in stock. Nobody likes being told what to buy. Even if you only have one product worth buying, have selection to show why that one is worth more than it is.

Address the cost last. Sell your product before the terms are negotiated. The price is set on a sliding scale, and you choose where it rests, often making it up on the spot: a collage of various contextual elements and largely governed by whim. Give trendsetters discounts and let your contact list look like the reservation roster at a Michelin-rated restaurant. Comp the people who'll sell for you without realizing it. Maintain marketing campaigns.

Always err on the side of the customer. Always go at least a point over weight. Complaints cost more than a bit of coke or crystal or calyx — they cost customers. Keep everyone happy.

These are my thoughts as I'm being trained in sales at the gym I've been attending since spring.

* * *

It's my fifth day of work, and if I knew how to fill out the sign-up sheets and where the business cards and trial passes were, I could be employee of the month. I could sell a broken water heater to a sun god. You doubt? Find a sun god who'll deny that.

On my second day I ran out of things to do and decided to tap a new market; I googled local psychotherapists and compiled a list:

Subject: Paying Wellness Forward

Hi Dr. [insert name],

My name's ██████ and I'm contacting you from ████████████ gym in ██████████.

    I was diagnosed several years ago with bipolar disorder (type 2) and have struggled with many of the issues that go hand in hand with that: substance abuse, relationship difficulties, inability to find work, and a social pariah status that ensures this list remains indefinite. I spent much of last winter in CAMH trying medication after medication, to no avail.

    Finally, in June, I signed up for a membership at the gym that I now work at. There were immediate improvements: better sleep, confidence, a network of staff dedicated to seeing my health improve; and as I stuck with it, longer term improvements: metabolic consistency, increased energy, and a sense that I was reaching a level of stability unimaginable at this time last year.

    I found ████████████████ especially helpful because it's not a chain. There's a non-judgmental attitude and a huge diversity in our members. Every time I come to work out (and now come to work) my spirits lift in a Pavlovian sort of response. It wasn't easy, but it was easier here than I thought possible.

I'm reaching out to you in this message because, in addition to it being my job, I am, fundamentally, a mental health advocate. I know how bad it can get, and how much just a few hours of exercise a week can help. I also know how intimidating it can be, as someone who suffers with MH issues, to start up at a gym. I want to help my community.

If you feel that this attitude and this facility is something your patients would benefit from, please put them into contact with me, and I would be more than happy to show them around, show them the ropes, and pay the wellness forward.

The regular membership rate is $99 registration and $69 per month (which includes a fitness consultation and a wide array of classes and programs), or $699 for a full year. The gym also provides child-minding services for busy parents.

I understand that for many patients this may be a bit of a stretch on the budget. Happily, there's a corporate promotion until January 15, which shaves the cost to $39 per month or $300 for a full year.

I hope this is of interest to you and your patients. I would love the opportunity to help those in need.

Kind regards,

██████

http://██████████.ca/

My supervisor had his doubts. He thought it was too long. Too much information. Not a hard enough sell. They wouldn't be interested, etc.

1)
Hi ████████,

Thank you for your email. I'm happy to hear how it's helped you and how passionate you feel. It's inspiring. I know first-hand how powerful exercise can be. It's not everything someone with MH challenges needs, but it offers a lot. I will definitely keep it in mind if my clients are looking for a gym, and I may even check it out myself! :)

████████

Sent from my iPhone

2)
Hi ████████. I will be glad to pass this on. Congratulations on your personal improvements and your articulate, encouraging openness.

    I wish you a happy holiday. Best, ████████

Sent from my iPhone

3)
Hi ████████,

Thanks for contacting us. We will definitely pass on this information to our team. Our Clinical Director, ████, also has another practice that's more focused on wellness and working with other practitioners with a holistic approach. I wonder if there's a

potential for some opportunities for collaboration
in the new year. If there's any interest on the part
of your management/team, let me know and I will
pass on your information to her as well.
Best Regards,

██████

Clinic Manager

4)
Hi ██████,
Thank you very much for your email and sharing
your inspirational story.

   I agree with your philosophy and am also an
advocate for whole person health, which includes
physical health, nutrition, and movement. The relationship between physical and emotional health
is significant and something I encourage clients to
deepen their connection with.

   I will certainly let clients know of the opportunity to join ███████████ to pursue their health
goals, and thank you for advising me of the promo- ·
tion, which would be very helpful.
All the best,

██████

    There were ten or so more like this, and they're still com-
ing in. No negative responses. I work on commission. The top
salesperson is quite impressed. He's the guy who signed me up.

FORTY
December 23, 2017

You may have noticed that I had mentioned a certain Chuckles Skullfucker earlier. What happened there?

We're moving into an apartment in the West End of Toronto in January. Right by High Park, near my family. Rushed? A bit, maybe, but we're close to help if we need it. Most likely rushed, really. We both admit it. We have no delusions about this, but we're both living in uncomfortable circumstances as it is (me with my family and her with hers, an hour's drive away), and it really does seem like the most practical solution. She's a very pragmatic person — not what you'd expect out of someone willing to date a bipolar with borderline.

We talk all day, every day. It's easy. Natural. Comfortable. She fits.

Apart from that I'm just working on wellness, my main priority, of which Chuckles is a major part. I'm exercising at the gym at least three times a week, sometimes up to five days, for at least an hour at a time. Intensive. I'm eating a bit better, too. Not ideally. But marginally.

The drugs? I'm mostly just on the decarboxylated honey oil now, but still occasionally eat some mushrooms or have a bit of MDMA. Never much. I don't need to lose it again. But I would love to get my hands on some acid.

FORTY-ONE
February 2018

I want Chuckles to get to know the psychedelic side of me. To that end, I've been taking steadily growing doses of mushrooms once every few months. I want her to know I can take them safely and be safe while I'm on them. And that I'm safe to be around while tripping. At 0.5 grams I was essentially microdosing: feeling very little and showing even less. At one gram I can tell that something is different, and smoking pot definitely increases the psychedelic vibes, but for all intents and purposes, I'm indistinguishable from your average law-abiding citizen. I could work. I could drive. At two grams I'm definitely feeling a bit looser, but Chuckles insists that she can barely tell a difference. Maybe I'm just odd to start with. So I decided to skip a few steps and jump to four grams.

Now, it's been a while since I took a substantial amount of a psychedelic, and you kind of forget a lot of what losing your mind entails when it's been this long. No matter how experienced you are, once you take some time off, it can feel almost new again. And while the psychedelic escapade-loving, ego death–seeking, oblivion-embracing version of me from university would scoff at a mere four grams of mushrooms, it is indeed a substantial dose. These particular mushrooms were Golden Teachers. Less visual. More entheogenic. More shamanistic. More connective to the world. They come by their name honestly.

I boiled a pot of water and waited a minute or two for it to cool down enough not to destroy the active ingredients. Pouring the water over an orange pekoe teabag (to mask to taste of mushrooms — think hay and manure combined with mildew) and a stainless steel tea steeper packed to the brim with four grams of powdered Golden Teachers, I stirred in a teaspoon of honey, squeezed a wedge of lemon into the mixture (to quicken my metabolism and enhance absorption), and waited several minutes.

Then I slammed it.

Within fifteen minutes I was feeling something, which was about fifteen minutes sooner than I'd expected using the tea method. This is usually indicative of a fairly powerful experience on the horizon, so I guess Chuckles will finally see me in a properly psychedelic state. I feel the trepidation typically associated with an oncoming life-altering experience. At least I have Chuckles with me.

I hope I don't scare the shit out of Chuckles.

"How ya feelin'?"

—I feel groovy. I feel … the groove. Grooving.

The thing about mushrooms is that your mind will construct the most insightfully simple, articulate, and creative statements you could imagine, far beyond the imaginative capacities of the sober, and you will desire desperately to share them with the world — to record, for posterity and the good of mankind, these nuggets of perfection. Then you will open your mouth.

—Umm, what?

"I said, 'How ya feelin'?'"

—If you were a soup, what soup would you be?

"Hahaha, um, well ... I guess, maybe mushroom soup? Or chicken soup? What sort of soup would you be?"

I have to think very, very, *very* hard.

—Ketchup. No, wait. Guacamole.

"Good lord. Are you OK?"

Chuckles has, essentially, no experience whatsoever with drugs. Like, none. Maybe not the best choice of sober-sitter, in retrospect. She'll have no way of determining what I'm experiencing. What level of ecstasy or fear I'm feeling. I decide to move closer, thinking that physical proximity equates to a level of psychic bonding.

Gradually, I trick myself. I actually do come to believe we share a consciousness, and I am immediately awash in a sweet warmth. Like a melted butterscotch blanket, the comfort of love's synchronicity strokes my central nervous system's core systemic processes. I turn to her to explain my new-found understanding.

—I, that is, *we*, because we are me, and you are I, and you can, right? You can?

"Mhmm?"

She strikes a look and raises an eyebrow, creating the impression of creasing her forehead into a series of crevasses etched into the glacial horizon of her frigid mindscape: Is she receding into the ice? Horror strikes. In the grips of my relational apotheosis, I understand myself as intrinsically linked to Chuckles, but tenuously hanging on by the unyielding threads of our uniqueness. If I think of us as *us*, instead of linked, as *me* or *I*, the whole construct of our being as one entity would collapse. If I recognize us as distinct and separate beings, it's over. Using the word *you* is off limits, lest the universe collapse on itself. She must be able to understand me. She must. Otherwise, I'm not right. Otherwise, none of this is right.

—We're. Me am, I mean, me, together forever, right? I. I. I'm I and so am we.

She looks perplexed. I point at her and say, "I." Then nod to get her to nod, then point at myself and say, "You." I work to get her to nod along, and with both of us nodding in unison I say, "Me." And when she says, "Us," I am horrified at the concept of separation. I then point back and forth between us and say, "Me. Me forever?"

"Mhmm. Gotcha. Forever."

There's no way she got that. But it was the right thing to say. And that says a lot about her.

FORTY-TWO

When should I finish this?

When has the story been told? Should I stop when I'm happy? Do I need to find "myself"? Or just keep going till it ends?

Do I wrap it up first? Or do I abandon it midstep?

Is it up to me?

FORTY-THREE

January 1, 2019, 1:30 a.m.-ish

The shawarma shop door slams open as snow swirls in around a clearly dome-blown character I'll be calling Actor. He grins vacantly and scans the group inside.

Two Palestinian dudes are manning the counter, frying falafels and making — swear to God — the best shawarma in the city; a younger guy, also Middle Eastern, is sitting alone, eyes blood red, nomming down a plate of chicken and assorted salads and sauces; and I'm sitting with Chuckles on barstools at a table coming out of the wall, trying to eat this piece of art without spilling a grain of rice or leaf of tabbouleh; next to us is a buddy from grade four I'll call Master for Dungeon

Master (yeah, I love D&D now — blame Chuckles, and he's a proper evil DM, always trying to kill your favourite character and whatnot). Chuckles and I had spent New Year's Eve at her cousin's apartment party, and it had been a good night, so I was in a good mood. And by this point I was pretty much sober — just trying to eat this sandwich.

Actor's eyes land on Chuckles. He looks at her like a prison inmate looking at a fresh fish. I do not approve.

"Let's see if you Canadians are as funny as everyone says you are. Hey, big guy, say something funny."

—Try the shawarma.

"That's fuckin' lame man. You're fuckin' lame."

He's clearly out of his mind. This guy's about 5'8", and maybe one hundred and sixty pounds. I'm 6'2" and two-fifty. He's not just drunk. He's on *something.*

"Hey, bro. We don't have to fight, bro. I'm just joking around. I just got in from BC — don't you recognize me?"

—I can honestly say that I don't.

"I'm a famous actor. I'm from Los Angeles. I have a manager."

—A lot of people have managers. And no, I still don't recognize you.

"Say, bro, you're not very nice. But your girlfriend is."

Here it comes.

"Why is she with you, bro? She's fit, bro. Why isn't she with me? You couldn't get her in your dreams. She should be coming home with me. What do you think of that, buddy, eh?"

I've pretty much just been swivelled around to look at this guy, sitting down, eating delicious shawarma. My neck is getting red, though, and I feel heat coming from my ears. Chuckles can tell the warning signs by now of when I'm getting upset, and she tries getting the attention of the shop workers to do something. They're paying close attention. The young guy sitting by himself (whom I'll call Peanut, for "Peanut Gallery"), eating a meal for a family of four, has taken an interest in the exchange and seems to be following the story through what I'd guess is a deep, deep indica stone.

—Why don't you ask her?

"See, bro, you can't even tell me. That's how bad she wants me."

I start looking around the restaurant, gauging where the security cameras are. Peanut pipes up.

"Bruv, that's mean."

"I didn't ask you, almond eyes."

"What the fuck? That's racist!"

Actor has turned back to me, having no time for Peanut.

"So, you think you could take me? You think you could beat me up and take her? Guy, look at your hair, man."

I'm just eating my sandwich.

Then I say something I probably shouldn't say.

—Don't fuck with me.

Actor's eyes are barely open, glazed over, and swaying rather than surveying.

"You think you're some sort of important guy? Big man's a big man? This is a Ukrainian neighbourhood. You know that? I have Ukrainian snipers training their scopes on you RIGHT NOW!"

Peanut is stuck on the last conversation. He addresses me.

"Bruv. Don't worry about him. I'll defend your girlfriend. She is beautiful."

What's with these guys? He addresses Actor:

"You wanna go, bruv? You wanna take this outside?"

Actor ignores him. All his attention is focused on securing Chuckles for himself.

"Did you know that I'm part of the Ukrainian mafia?"

—I thought you were an actor from LA? Is there much crossover? And yes, I know this is a Ukrainian neighbourhood. I grew up in it.

Then on a whim, I decide to see what will happen if I say some words from various Slavic languages and make it look like a sentence.

—*Dobry dzień, DakhaBrakha, na zdoròv'je.*

All I've said is "good day" in Polish, named a Ukrainian folk band, and said "you're welcome" in Russian, but something seems to have been triggered in his basic biological survival instincts.

"So *you* have the snipers."

Sure. I can run with this.

—Bang on, motherfucker.

At this point I finish my sandwich and stand up, to reinforce the full impact of the situation Actor has gotten himself into. My shadow envelops him. I have a knife in my back pocket, but I know those can get you in more trouble than you should get into over a ruined sandwich experience. Just in case, I grab a plastic knife, very subtly, and slide it up my sleeve. I also have a short umbrella that sort of shoots out about a foot when you press a button.

"So what, bro, you're gonna blow my brains out instead of giving me your girl? You're gonna shoot me over some bitch? My manager will fuck you up, bro. You ain't got shit, homie. Look at your clothes, guy. Your hair bun is so 2017."

I think all of us aside from Actor pull a double take at that. Peanut pokes in again.

"Bruv, that was like a year and two hours ago."

Actor is beyond reasoning.

"Your girl should be mine. Hey, don't you wanna come with me?"

Chuckles breaks her silence.

"Dude, do you think you're still at the club? We're in a fucking sandwich shop. Listen, we're just trying to get past you to go home. So please, just get the fuck out of the way."

He doesn't take kindly to her tone:

"Shut the fuck up, princess. Nobody asked you."

At this point, after Chuckles had made motions and hand gestures, the shopkeepers are calling the police. She's shaking. She isn't used to this sort of encounter, and she knows my past. She's looking for a way out, for both of us: holding on to the back of my shirt both to remind me that she's here with me and to dissuade me from charging the creep. I know that, but I lose my shit anyway.

Having scoped out the locations of the security cameras, I know I'm in the clear; the one opposite me was obscured by Actor. I untuck the white plastic knife, find the sharpest, hardest part, and bring it with professional speed to his throat. He hadn't seen any of this, he doesn't realize it's plastic. I also lift him with my left arm and slam him against the wall, pinning him several inches above the ground. He barely flinches.

"Gonna kill me, bro? Gonna stab me for your girl? Gonna radio some Uki mobsters to pump me up?"

I'm not reaching this guy very well.

—Fuck you, waste of a sandwich.

I point the tip of my umbrella at him, press the button, and shit-hit him right in the solar plexus; then I keep pinning him against the wall while I motion for Chuckles and

Master to leave ahead of me. I can hear sirens. I stage-whisper to Chuckles:

—Reach into my pocket and get rid of the knife.

She deftly plucks my knife out and stows it in her bag. She should be a pickpocket. At this point the shopkeepers have come out from behind the counter. They're urging us out. Mostly, I'm guessing, because they don't want to be a murder-scene restaurant, but just after we leave, and before Actor does, they lock the door.

Scurrying down the street, we see the police converge on the location. The icy walk home is fraught with fears of being pulled over and frisked. But a month went by and nothing happened. I visited the shop for my sought-after shawarma, and to my surprise, the shop owners were elated to see me, yelling "That's the guy!" and pointing me out to the other employees. They comped my meal and thanked me for ridding them of "the troublemaker." When I asked what had happened, they said he was arrested. I guess he never made it as an actor.

FORTY-FOUR
Late 2018

Chuckles and I haven't spent a day apart since we moved in together. We're stuck. Both in the good and bad senses. We depend on each other to an unhealthy amount. We're each other's "safety." And we both know we'd be lost if something were to happen.

On June 30, 2018, the eve of Canada Day, I took a trip out to trip out in High Park with Smurf, of CAMH escape fame. He'd gone through the jail experience, too, now. Broke his hand on the wall. Guess he had it in him. He didn't really catch much in the way of repercussions. I'm still not clear on the details, and he's not keen to talk about it. Understandable.

He's on the path to … enlightenment? Debatable, but he's better off than me; he's got a path. He's training to be a yogi (bear ... sorry, I can't help myself). He's a full-blown hippie: drum circles, ecstatic dance, shamanic mushroom rituals, etc. But he seems like he's doing well. He makes enough money to live comfortably and do yoga all day, more hippie shit all night, and a whackload of psychedelic drugs. What a life. He's even gotten into the whole Ayurvedic cooking thing, and I must say his food is tasty as all hell. I can't deny that something about his life appeals.

I've always wanted to move out to the middle of nowhere, where land is cheap, with a few close friends: we'd buy up adjoining plots of land and create an artist commune/stopping point on the hippie trail. Live in an eco-anarcho/communist utopia within the larger, safer confines of socialist Canada, which can actually defend us hippies with, like, guns and soldiers and supersonic jets and satellites and shit. It sounds perfect. I could write, draw, grow my gardens, live in an Earthship hobbit-hole, and be an *artiste* gentleman-farmer. Raise my kids like humans. Fuck yeah.

Smurf met me next to a parking lot in the park at about ten in the morning, under a tree where he had a blanket out and was doing inhuman stretching postures for his own well-being, but also, I suspect, for the entertainment of passersby. He's rail thin. Classic yogi look. Hasn't showered in a week and only uses essential oils when he does. "My natural oils are the best for me." He's wearing a mishmash of globalized, culturally appropriated clothing — all hippie brand, but all purchased first-hand. He rolls his own *Nicotiana rustica* cigarettes, and in the back of his car is a replica of Bilbo's sword, Sting, a battle-ready claymore, and a plash palatka: "It's good for all sorts of stuff; you can use it as a tent, a cloak, or in the apocalypse."

One time Chuckles, Smurf, and I were playing D&D. It was his turn to be the Dungeon Master, and he had something special in store for us. We prepared our characters with care: the first thing he had us do was take off all of our clothing and drop our weapons and go on a journey of self-discovery. The only enemies we encountered turned out to be mirrors of ourselves who would only attack when they were attacked themselves. We made peace when we hugged them and "accepted ourselves."

Fucking hippies.

He rolled up his blanket with care and put it into his larger trip bag … stuffed for any (well, most any) eventuality. We sat down in the shade as it was incendiary outside. It felt like there was a forest fire not far away and the wind was gusting hot, damp air at us.

He pulled out of his bag a few small vials full of brown powder and an ornate little pipe device, then he got me to try something called rapé (pronounced "hepé"), which is a type of tobacco-based snuff (with different other herbs, producing the various vials he had) you actually shoot up your nostrils with the South American–inspired decorative blow-pipe I wish I'd known about back when I still did cocaine. It was my first time. It burned like only the fire of human thought can. Smurf said with a sense of superiority:

"It hurts less the more you do, and it hurts a lot if you used to put a lot of bad stuff up there."

Ahhh, fuck off, Big Poppa Smurf. I didn't really notice anything, especially after his claims that it was a revelatory drug with deep shamanic roots.

We found our way to a quiet little clearing surrounded by fallen trees and vines, shadowy patches and small clearings awash in dew speckles. We were on a hill that rollicked gently in parts and dropped off a little steeper in others, with a muddy path down to the pond's edge. The bugs were out in force. Bugs bother me when I'm sober. Once you start tripping, your priorities change. We were there by about eleven in the morning, and it started to get more than just pretty hot. Humid to the point of choking. I'd already drunk through half my water.

Smurf led the way in a bit of yogic breathing practice. In through one nostril, out through the other, back in with the second, then out with the first; repeat ad nauseam type thing. I was getting restless. I wasn't really focusing on the breathing or the meditative aspects all that much. I was antsy to get on with the day. The pond looked inviting as all hell on this hot-ass day. It was tranquil, with little frogs hopping and fish swimming and a tree half-fallen into the water, supporting a mini ecosystem. There were lily pads and ducklings paddling around, dipping under the water now and then, popping up with beaks full of algae.

—So ... do you wanna do this or what?

"So impatient. Tsk tsk. Let's wait. I prefer to do it in the evening. There are more visuals, and they're more intricate. The night holds mystery. The rhythms of the moon, secrets of the stars, and other things."

I don't want to wait in this little grove for the ten or so hours it'll take to get dark.

—I'm more of a daytime person. It immerses you more in reality that way. What is really appears as it is, y'know?

"I suppose I could try it. But this will likely be a strange one."

He giggled, mostly to himself, in his weird yogi giggle.

Then uhh ... umm ... err ... I did something a bit silly. He pulled out the LSD. I hadn't had any in ages ... and ached for reconnection with that mode of thought. That sheer artfulness of hue the universe takes on under the influence of this miracle molecule is beyond enticing to someone enamoured by the strange, paradoxical, and logically illogical. Unwrapping the crinkly aluminum less than inconspicuously as tourists wandered the paths around us, he showed me four little teal-blue squares of paper with swirl patterns on them ... It's always swirls with LSD. It's a very swirly drug. Natural logarithmic spirals blast off in every direction and appear in everything. Sacred geometry, indeed.

Smurf and I were alone. Chuckles had stayed at home, having seen me on mushrooms and assuming I was fine with the yogi (bear) monitoring me. I'd left telling her I was going to keep it to a half, or one at most ... not wanting to dive headfirst back into a chemical I hadn't had in a while. Acid is a lot more hectic, frantic, frenetic, energetic than mushrooms or mescaline. It has almost an amphetamine quality of energy. This is good for picking up your spirits and generally steering clear of super bad trips most of the time, unlike mushrooms, which generally have a fairly sedentary nature (and, for me, are more likely to produce more common bad trips) ... but it means that when an LSD trip goes bad. Well. Yeah ...

Smurf took two of the four tabs and put them on his tongue.

"So, uhh ... how do you wanna do this? I don't have scissors, so we could just rip one in half?"

I took the other two tabs and stuck them up into my gums.

"Oh shit. Goodness, it's gonna be like that, eh?"

I mean, I've taken ten thousand micrograms of LSD before, so I was fairly confident about the two-hundred-microgram tabs Smurf had acquired … if they even were that dose, y'know? No taste this time. So far so good. I had a big bottle now half full of water, since it was about thirty-one degrees Celsius and I take lithium, for which you're supposed to drink a lot of water. As a molecule, lithium carbonate is basically just a salt. Stay hydrated or weird shit happens.

You can see where I'm going here.

After about thirty minutes I felt an intense rush of energy and excitement. A feeling I wasn't expecting for another half hour, or so. This, generally, meant I was in for some shit.

—I feel it already.

"Well. That's something, isn't it now."

Then I heard that textbook, self-assured hippie giggle of psychic infirmity. Fuck you, dude.

* * *

There's a thick cloud of gnats above me, Rorschaching to the remnants of breeze pushed under our bush clearing's canopy. Smurf squats on a thick mat of leaves as he self-administers bowl after bowl of rapé, alternating nostrils between hollow-cheeked huffs of Jack Herer in a semi-controlled exerciseperiment of entropy. Ants arc all over my twisting torso as I'm trapped in the forty-degree-after-humidity sweat sticking me to my T-shirt. This feels so fucking goo. I stand up from the anthill archipelago I'm sprawled over and begin exploring the contents and edges of our clearing. I focus very closely on the bark of a tree and see it growing in very, very, verrry slow motion, with bugs glittering in the crevices and crawling

along in pheromonal, preordained paths, like blood vessels
across the surface of the flora. Greenery is in more than just
the lush leaves and grasses and weeds; it permeates the air, the
pond, the pale skin of Smurf. Every imaginable shade of green.
Unimaginable shades of green, too. Infinite greens ... let alone
the separate, but lesser, infinities of yellows, browns, maroons,
oranges, etc. Green is my favourite colour. Green swirls are
my favourite visual pattern. The LSD is alive, and I'm in the
midst of an infection of perfection. There are echoes in the
open spaces all around us. I test these echoes and begin speaking to the Garden of Eden I'm breathing in, mixed with the
herbal aroma of the vividly alive plants all around us and the
piney smell of burning Jack Herer. The echoes are dynamic.
I can sense the difference in time between the echoes of each
individual branch, each leaf, each cell, each atom. Sounds surround me in exponential pluralities, rocketing off into eternity
at an expanding warp speed, like a steep parabola on either side
of my y-axis. I wonder what poetry would sound like.

—Do not go gentle into that good night.

Do not be gentle when confronting that good night.

—That good night is not gentle to go into.

Is the night even good?

—Do not go gentle into that foul day.

Accept that a day can be a foul day.

—Accept the foul day in a leap of faith.

Become Kierkegaard's knight of faith.

—Accept that night.

But not today.

—I can taste the haste with which I wish to paste my perfect thoughts on the face of the planet so as not to waste the
beautiful grace with which they were created; like the invention

of infomercial-intended serrated knives that can cut through cans with no effort, just as an expert swordsman's katana can. Man, I can rhyme, winding my way round a boast like a grape-wine vine round a post, I make the most of the language I know, and my breath flows naturally with wind as it blows. I WANNA LICK MY FUCKIN' ELBOWS! Phew. Fuck me. FUCK ME SIDEWAYS WITH A SLEDGEHAMMER!

Not my finest work. But I feel a wave of incipient creativity. I want to paint. I want to act. I want to dance. I want to bake word soup and play the banjo. I don't know how to play the banjo, but something tells me I can learn how *right now*.

"Whoa, man. Easy there."

—Hahahaha. I'm having too much fun.

* * *

One thing about psychedelics — classical tryptamines, mostly — is that they make me feel like a kid again, at least in the first of three stages. I want to play. Play is *very* important. Playtime consumes all. And I get the giggles. Overwhelming giggles. Like, I don't know why I'm giggling, then I giggle about that, then I giggle because I think I'm broken, and eventually I'm giggling so hard it's getting difficult to breathe. So, good for a raucous laugh, all in all. Then I get very animated and excitable. I want to do things. FUN THINGS! Things I haven't done in a long time or wasn't allowed to do. I wanna play with cars and Barbies, make couch forts, chew on blankets. These are very common, if not universal, themes. THOU ART TODDLER. The most commonplace event seems overwhelmingly profound and unusual. There is a sense of novelty to absolutely *everything*.

I might as well mention the functions and parameters of the next two stages of the classic tryptamine experience. Stage two is the proper *psychedelic* element. This is where the stereotypical "my mind is blown" or "tripping mad balls" lives. The visual content is most pronounced in the second stage, and the mental faculties are just absolutely shot. Neurons are far too fried out to make sense of anything. But you might just surprise yourself. You'll remember forgotten memories or find things you thought you'd lost. You'll think of old problems in new ways and can come up with ingenious solutions to stymying issues. Man, that's what Israel and Palestine need, a mescaline trip together ...

The third phase is reintegration, when I like to do most of my art. The "real" world is coming back, and you're just trying to hold on to the fleeting memories of the psychedelic experience. You're tired, but the ass-kicking you just took keeps you going to gradually acclimatize to the world as the normals see it.

Then it's over.

Well, not really. A psychedelic experience changes you. Permanently. And even just a small amount can physiologically boost your mood over the course of several weeks ... so it has some staying power.

* * *

Anyhow, I was getting to the point where I was tripping over roots and losing the ability to catch myself before I landed. I was higher than I'd expected. Beauty.

I meandered over to Smurf and lay down with my head on my backpack, staring up through the canopy of leaves at the contortionist clouds.

Smurf handed me the cheap steel pipe, and I didn't really think about it. Second nature.

I accepted a proffered puff, took what I thought was probably just enough to boost the Lucy's edge, and passed it back. Jack Herer is a very energetic strain of sativa. More like a cup of coffee than cannabis, in my mind. It doesn't take long before Smurf seems like a spirit guardian, assuming beast form of half man/half some-sort-of-goat-creature and ancestral lineage to a more shamanistic, animistic origin. His advice seemed of paramount importance. As the weed took effect, I heard his words, seemingly repeated ad infinitum, though likely I was just stuck in a time loop:

"Lie down, and breathe. Focus on the breath. It's all about the breath. Breath is life."

Lying down in synchronicity to the exhale, I felt myself fold through the forest floor into the far, far, far away from escape.

My vision was rolling along at however many frames per second on an old-school film reel. It started splicing in odd visions every few milliseconds. Then it started splicing in more. Soon reality and a parade of alternate realities were meandering away in front of my eyes like a View-Master toy that had somehow incongruously incorporated the grove I was in, with Smurf, as well as hundreds of varied scenes populated by strangers, friends, family, enemies, aliens, and shadows of angelic proportions. The film roll began running at odd speeds. My eyes had fallen out of synchronicity with each other. One would be watching *Singin' in the Rain* and one would be watching the terraforming of Enceladus, while my internal visual monitor was trying to pierce these pictographs of madness to find the anchor of Smurf. *Let's get back to that breathing exercise.* I felt like I could benefit from it. I felt like I might need it a bit. Finally, the film roll began to flicker and sputter. It bubbled. A small flame broke out in the pictures on the bottom left of my vision and progressed to the top right in an amoebic movement. All I saw was the light from the projector and the occasional faint overlay of a ... a something.

I began thinking of things greater than myself. What I believe in. Who I am. What the world owes me and what I owe the world.

I believe in anarchy, that is — philologically — a voluntary and participatory system of philosophically self-governing society ...

My moral autonomy is not ordinary; no, normally — in the excess of economically repressed, socially regressive, and depressingly oppressed global territories that constitute the disproportional majority — my conformity would be as mandatory as subscribing to the stereotypes entrenched in antiquated Disney princess stories. This makes me part of an improbably privileged minority. Note that my good fortune is not a right; it's as right as those historically recorded notes of hometown heroes' valour in vanquishing uncivilized, foreign vermin that serve as vindication for vicious and invalid, vile victories, and the accompanying, ad hoc homilies. It's as glorious as any unremembered acts of aggression that ask for atrocities to be committed against equally complex manifestations of causality in psycho-biochemistry — or the so-stamped "enemy."

I, through happenstance — not destiny — have been granted what some would call "God-given" opportunities to evolve beyond the heteronomously handed-down hypocrisies, termed *social policies*, that split the planet into polities on nominal bases (like phenotypy or theology), and which pit these arbitrarily established, post-colonial "countries" into endless poverty and self-defeating enmity — I can study, I can read, and I can teach: freely.

I must develop as anomalous and destroy the dominant doctrine of dichotomy between master and slave mentalities. How? Simply ...

Exercise my rational faculties of sanity and exorcise the fictional mythology that feeds my vanities. Pull myself into a perpetual sense of the present tense. Become aware of the stairs that I'm tearing up; care that I am ever on the verge of becoming but have never conceived of just being. Because every step I am speeding through represents a plateau that I have just failed to appreciate. Please, I must try to perceive a piece of peace unique to myself in this set and setting. I only get what I'm for when I forget what I'm getting, and I forget what I'm for when I only get getting more. Got it?

Harmony is achieved where the declining line of quantity meets the rising tide of quality, colliding like this point in time's designed to be and finally divining itself definably as mass amassing energy and no longer hiding quietly inside of ... me.

I see that I am wise, alive, and free.

I now recognize reality as a shared, subjective, experiential entity that's purposefully playing impossibly complex games of chess against itself from a concurrently conscious multiplicity of personalities in an infinite eternity of specificity mixed with general relativity, heavily held in rapid revolution 'round a heavenly, illusory, gravitational pseudo-psyche-spirit-university gripped in solipsistic self-discovery. And now I'm finally thinking, "I am *fucking crazy*." But I'm not. To ask after the method in madness is to misunderstand my meaning of seeking reason. And to me, even reality's fleeting.

To paraphrase a great poem I don't know the writer of, and which may not actually exist, "I fell into it like a daydream, or a fever." I was literally illiterate when it came to time. A curious body-load sensation spiralled my head up and to the side, and I was reminded horribly of Java's twisted-neck smile. I tried to shake off that thought and shook off more than I thought thought could take. Ego death and coagulated eternities had an illegal, underground dance party, and I was the only participant invited to this horror-filled lack-of-light show. I dipped in and out of consciousness like an ice cream cone being adorned in various coatings. Each time I came out, reality was different. Hey, look, sparkles! Hey, look, a nihilistic expanse of time-defying evil portents in a landscape defined by its lack of definition!

The geometry of 8A and B can shove some baroque- and rococo-inspired fucking pixelated neo-virtual firecrackers up their asses with the intensity of what was going on in my made-to-find-meat-and-nuts-and-fire-and-shelter-and-mates mind. I, a lowly and simpering *Homo sapiens sapiens*, brought low by the dazzling stupidity of my own actions and the intensity of my supercharged synapses doing the neurological equivalent of shooting blanks at a beyond *beyond* beyondness. Beyond human. Beyond alien. Beyond being. Beyond reality. Beyond *reality*.

I felt a super prenatal goddess presence and all-around judgment. I wondered how I measure up as a human, given who I am, what I've done, etc. How will I be judged? What if, at the moment of death, you're presented with realistic depictions of all the people you've harmed and lied to, and you have to come clean to them, not knowing whether this is really an exercise in soul cleansing, a test from the transdimensional entities, or

you're tripping and just think you're dying, and you legitimately are coming clean to these people who hate you (or should).

I thought of my ex, Teddy, Dillon, Keeper, Lorax, María,
Tania, Eddie, Innocent, Needle, Pole, and Skittles — even Frat
Boy, Soulless, Sheng, Leprechaun, Granny, and Xerxes ... I
was so sorry. I was sorry I was in their lives. I was sorry I was
in anyone's life. I was sorry that truth is subjective. I was sorry,
too, to the First Man, Big Poppa Smurf, Chud, my parents,
my family at large, and Chuckles Skullfucker. My self-disgust
extended to them. I shouldn't be in any of their lives. I saw
them all around me as Venetian masks interchanging between
phantasmal grey-white cloaks. They towered above me in judgment. There were too many to count. I've hurt so many people.
I will hurt so many more.

I kept taking a huge breath, then exhaling it as slowly and
purposefully as possible until my lungs were almost deflated,
then holding it for as long as possible. Each breath felt like a
failure. Each breath felt like gravity dragging me back to this
void of creation. Each breath kept me stuck in this horrible
exercise of all-consuming mindfulness. Each breath sucked me
up more into this wretched business of "living." If this life was
reality, it was unacceptable, it was horrifying. I had to reach the
real *reality*. I've also been told since then that I was shouting
how thirsty I was. This makes sense, spending hours sweating
shitloads of LSD out of every pore on the hottest day of the
year with nowhere enough water to sustain myself. I remember
my throat felt like it was closing; I was so thirsty. My lips were
sticky. My mouth was slimy. I was parched, and right next to
all that water. Thirsty enough to try my hand at drowning.

I took a lot from this experience. I learned that I'm willing to
go the full mile for reality. I came to believe that I couldn't get

back unless I mastered myself to the point I could control my breathing into ceasing. So when it proved challenging because, well, it's physically impossible to stop yourself breathing with will alone, I eventually charged into Grenadier Pond to inhale the water, just to get back to reality. After all, "Breath is life."

At the moment I no longer recalled breathing air, I had a flash of the most curious sort. I had the distinct impression that I was a little girl, planting rice in a paddy in East Asia, sometime in the Middle Ages. I was being reincarnated, and it would be wretched. I would be a literal wretch. I hadn't thought that you could reincarnate backwards in time. That's atrocious. Think of all the misery experienced by our ancestors, and by the vast majority of living humans. Somehow, digging into a past-life regression (of this life), I knew this was a turbulent time in East Asia ... I worried momentarily about the Mongols. Reincarnation seems horrible.

Suddenly I was brought back to a semi-semblance of reality, still being strobed by intense fits of psychosis, and totally unable to discern or determine what was going on. I remember rolling down the hill ... kinda. I remember being wrestled out of the water by a group of people. I remember other people watching. People with dogs. Tourists. People with cameras. Then I remember lying sideways and being rolled down a path and looking at Chuckles and thinking, *When did she get here?* Then: *Fuck. I ruined it.* I learned later that Smurf had called her when he saw things going downhill for me and she hustled on over in terror.

I remember parts of being in the ambulance, tied down. Parts of being in emergency, tied down. Parts of seeing my parents while in a chemical frenzy of confusion and sensitivity ... still tied down.

I later learned I'd made a potentially fatal mistake. I hadn't looked up the contraindications of my new medicines. Lithium is strictly off limits when using classic tryptamines, or most psychedelics for that matter. I'd had small amounts of mushrooms since starting lithium, most notably the four-gram trip to show Chuckles I was chill on psychs, and I suppose those *had* been a bit more intense than usual. But I hadn't had a big, big, big dose until that Canada Day eve.

The mixture was horrific. Definitely a contender for my worst trip experience. Probably the winner, given the results. For days afterward I was having seizures, aftershocks from the seismic activity my body had presented while mid-cataclysm.

What follows is the account rendered to me by Chuckles Skullfucker. I have next to no memory of it.

* * *

In the little bend where the pond met the path about ten people had gathered to watch Smurf and another onlooker struggle with my writhing, aspiring corpse, which was performing crocodilian death spins while Smurf dove under to keep my head above the water. I twisted and squirmed like a sea snake in an effort to dunk my head back under, simply wanting to drink. Chuckles was on the phone with 911, which Smurf had called before chucking the phone to Chuckles and chasing after me into the pond.

After the violent struggle, once they managed to drag me back onto solid ground, I lay squealing in high-pitched moans and gasping sounds. I was choking myself. When the cops finally arrived — they'd gotten lost in the park — they refused to give me mouth-to-mouth since I'd been in the pond and they didn't want to endanger me. Instead, they tied me to a stretcher, still making no eye contact, and wheeled me, screaming/gasping for air, into an ambulance.

To onlookers, I had fought with another tripping yogi (bear), a group of cops, and eventually the paramedics, all while aspirating pond scum and rolling down a hill of thorns and branches. Must've been a sight. Smurf took a video. I hope it's not loose.

Smurf and Chuckles walked behind, and off I went. They weren't even sure which hospital I was headed to. Since Chuckles and I were still fresh together, she didn't have my parents' phone number and had to reach out to my sister to connect with my folks.

"Is everything OK?"

"Should be, yep."

Chuckles tried my parents, but they were out with the festivities. She started crying uncontrollably. An intensely still-tripping Smurf tried to console her, to little effect.

Chuckles and Smurf eventually decided to go wait for my parents outside their house, on their fancy street — Chuckles continuing to make frantic calls and Smurf striking a pose and returning to his rapé … looking super sketchy, as usual.

This having little effect, they took a cab to the local hospital (and the most likely place I'd eventually wind up), Smurf still soaked in pond scum. There they found me.

I wanted to give Chuckles a kiss for comfort, but I was a biohazard, so Chuckles refused. It hurt. I just couldn't understand.

I was kept in isolation until I was untied from my straps and led down the hall for a shower (hose down), first with intensely cold, then intensely hot water. It didn't feel great on the dangling flaps of skin hanging off my raw kneecaps. I was led back to a bed. I can't remember if I was tied up again. Chuckles and Smurf took the momentary reprieve to go get something to eat, at which point my parents arrived.

Apparently, when they came into the room, I popped up in bed and acted almost sober. Positive, outgoing. Perhaps this was the drugs, or perhaps it was a deep, underlying fear of the disappointment my parents would feel if they knew I'd slipped up again. But they already knew. They were pissed. They called me an idiot and left. That was that.

My clothes were ruined. My shoes, it goes without saying, were garbage. I smelled like sewage for the next few days. I was confused as to what had happened. Nobody really filled me in. I was apologetic. I knew I'd done something wrong ... but I couldn't tell what, aside from the freak-out. I didn't really think about how much I'd made people worry.

Chuckles was mad at me for taking more than I'd said I would. That was understandable. I was caught up in the moment and stupid, and I have to pay for that. But I think she recognized that I was suffering enough already. She didn't rub it in.

She confided to me months later that I sometimes get a certain look in my eye that makes her think it might happen again. I may just break and go feral anytime. She says it took months to feel comfortable again. I believe it.

When we finally spoke to my folks again, we went to their house to try to have a civilized talk. My mom said that they thought maybe they couldn't trust me anymore, and that maybe I should return the keys to their house. That was a breakup motion, to me.

I cut off contact from my family. Completely. Possibly forever. I stopped returning their calls. I instructed my psychiatrist not to talk to them. I avoided them in public. I became afraid of going outside for fear of one of them seeing me and doing ... God knows what. I fell into true paranoia. I felt they were after me — they were a powerful family, and they were after me. I threatened my dad with a restraining order.

One time we saw my dad and sister together on Bloor Street West. They had my youngest nephew in a stroller. They saw me. I panicked and led Chuckles into the subway with me. We got on a train to nowhere to hide, me sweating profusely, under the impression they were following.

God, that hurts.

I plotted my revenge.

FORTY-FIVE
2002-2018

How do you "normals" do it? Without drugs, I mean. Like, I see the kids studying, which I can make sense of doing sober, even if I don't, but then they go home and just … like … don't do anything new. They don't explore. They don't push boundaries. They are comfortable with where the walls sit and the proportions on their plate and the way their feet balance them on the floor. What the fuck?

I am soooooooooo bored. All the time.

How does one stay away from boredom? Especially since tolerance builds up quickly. Nobody wants to waste a precious tab of acid or become a heroin addict. So I had a sort of schedule throughout high school and university … and at a few select other times. Knowing that all the classic tryptamines — psilocybin, LSD, and mescaline — have a cross-tolerance, and it lasts almost two weeks, makes it hard to "keep up with the trip."

That is, until you get your fingers mucky in chemistry and the underworld. There are plenty of non-classic psychedelics, plus narcotics, and a few one-offs. I tried, as responsibly as possible, to set up a schedule. At least a week between classic tryptamines: coke day, ope day, K day, molly day, benzo day, amphetamine day, experimental molecule day, smokin' DMT all day (still a classic tryptamine but better, because you can smoke it time after time), etc. And always, gargantuan amounts of cannabis. At least seven grams a day just for myself, most as poppers. If you don't know what they are, you're about to crave one. It's as close as cannabis comes to crack. It's usually a make-shift bong with a glass stem. Tobacco is packed in the tip, then covered with anything else (usually just cannabis, but we'd add all sorts of concentrates and chemicals), then "popped" through after lighting. They fuck you up something stupid, but your lungs will be Swiss cheese in weeks.

Anyway, kids, the point is, you can be fucked up forever; just keep your horizons open. The internet is your friend, but take a reasonable sample size of trip reports before risking any-thing. I was part of the generation just before this. When I was handed a pill, I took the pill … or two.

At least by 2018 my guy knows exactly what's in the stuff he sells me from the Rainbow Collective (a.k.a. the hippie mafia). Because I know I'll still be in this scene for a while. It's a life.

You "normals" may well be asking by now how we do it. Honestly, dunno. It's gotta catch up to me, though.

FORTY-SIX
Early 2018

Chuckles has expressed interest ... very rudimentary interest ... in psilocybin mushrooms. Obviously, due to her health anxieties, we'd try by dipping her finger in some flakes and eating those to make sure she's not allergic, but hopefully we'd be able to go further than that.

I feel like a pusher when I talk about psychedelics. I do love them, but also fear and respect them.

I'm excited for Chuckles. I know the first few doses, as we gradually go from 0.25 grams to 0.5 to 0.75 to one gram, etc. (with two weeks between each test), will be slow, but I'm excited vicariously. I remember my first experience. It was life-changing.

I know there's been postulation that the psychedelic experience is one of the key hallmarks of humanity. Along a lifeline, there are numerous possible defining moments: love, death (both yours and others'), self-realization, childbirth, aging, going mad, killing, etc. The postulation is that the psychedelic experience is no different, in that it is an action or experience from which there is no return and that changes the subject. I wouldn't disagree. I've been in love, survived deadly situations, been locked up in prison (albeit briefly) and psychiatric institutions, and travelled widely, but I still find psychedelics to be something definitively *else*. They return me to childhood and its open-eyed wonder but also allow me to psychically walk the surface of infinite suns across endless expanses and eras and cosmos, and to acquire with them a specific "wisdom" that feels both eternal and divine.

I consider psychedelics to be one of the five to ten or so things that define a human experience. You might as well give it a go if you're interested in yourself and the things your mind does. But take caution. The dose makes the poison.

I'm still terrified of Chuckles having a bad trip. She's different from the strangers I trip-sit for. Hence the extra care. The one thing I would never wish upon anyone is a negative psychedelic experience, or a full-blown psychotic episode …

FORTY-SEVEN
July 2019

What am I doing? Legit question. I could ask myself that. I'm living off of leftovers. I haven't spoken to my family in a year, and I'm facing eviction. I'm trying to write this and generally failing, slowly. And autocorrect for some reason wants to change *failing* to *falling*. Just noting.

Really. I'm waiting. No clue what for. Magic? The right word? Might as well be. I don't like my names, except my family name, which feels ironic right now. I study a lot, in strange ways. I don't necessarily read much, except the news, but I do the podcast thing, tons of YouTube info-farming. I'm reinforcing my childhood interests in history and philosophy and art and science that university, college, and the CanLit community robbed me of.

I'm also learning more about myself and the psychiatric processes that go into me being me. I've learned that, while displaying a lot of borderline personality disorder traits, since there's so much crossover between borderline and bipolar, the fact that I have bipolar disorder overrides the diagnosis of BPD. My doctor has also determined that I'm bipolar type 1, not 2. What all of this tells me is unclear since nothing has changed. The phrasing seems to constantly be mutating in psychiatry, but the object of description remains relatively steadfast. Regardless, it's helpful when describing my condition to strangers ... just say the diagnosis and they google it, then decide whether you're worth the trouble. Is that getting closer to the meaning of a *true* name? A total baring of the soul with every introduction?

I draw my comics, too. Dark, twisted comics. It seems more straightforward to just visually blast an image and short phrase into someone's temporal lobes and prefrontal cortex rather than expect them to read a whole weird-ass poem or memoir. It's straight efficiency. It's going nowhere on Instagram; I don't get the technology or the strategies, or I'm just not up to it. #anti-social. Good for a laugh, though.

I am, however, back to writing this for the moment — which is pleasant and feels like a huge accomplishment. I haven't written or read in more than a year (gasp if you must), and I've written the last four chapters or so in three or four nights! Woot! Though, I realize, at thirty, that I need reading glasses. The first draft of this chapter looked like a redcoat slaughter on a snowy field before the edit.

FORTY-EIGHT
Retrospective on 2009

I fucking love freestyling. I can't anymore, but once upon a time.

It came out of nowhere. It mixed a burgeoning intellect with competitiveness, dynamism, a bit of good old-fashioned cockiness, and most importantly, the mode of thought that eventually morphed into poetry, then prose, then comics, this writing, and even casual conversation. To think in metaphor and simile and rhyme and symbology and slanted approaches is a lesson far more valuable than most of my formal education. Plus, I was selling a shitload of drugs … so recklessness and braggadocio was aplenty. And I had the street cred to back up my freestyling boasts, which was rare.

My brother-in-law once bought me a book of hip-hop song lyrics, presented as poems. It's true. Established "print writers" might condescend to hip hop, or spoken word, but that's more a failing of imagination on their parts than a failing in the qualitative properties of the art forms. The ideas (some good, some bad, some genius, and some you've deluded yourself in your mania into believing are heaven-sent) are intrusive. They never stop. They're impermanent by nature, even between planning and putting pen to the page, they change. They come at night and haunt you with their possible disappearance before being recorded. A pen and pad become as necessary as an Ativan in a mental ward. The thoughts won't go away. The writing is a sort of disease, if not a symptom of an underlying illness. Losing a thought to the flood of inspiration or the fog of depression feels like an intellectual miscarriage, but no sooner can you mourn it than another needs attention. I have this persistent belief that everything must be recorded and stored for posterity, as if the summation of my writing holds some sort of psychic magic, like the spell of a life incarnate.

Is *writing* magic?

FORTY-NINE

Spring 2020

Something that feels good — magical, even — is my life. Weird, I know, especially close to the end of this story. But in all seriousness, it's getting better every day. I have Chuckles, and I'm making inroads back to my family. I reconnected with my grandma, first. I needed to see my grandpa: as his Parkinson's progresses, there's only so much time. And I couldn't leave him. I realized quickly how lonely my grandma was and endeavoured to spend more time with both of them. So Chuckles and I see them almost weekly now. Even more amazingly, I've met up with my dad — under the supervision of my psychiatrist (for safety), and after they'd had several sessions alone together getting my dad to understand my diagnoses and their ramifications.

This happy circumstance largely came by way of Chuckles having somewhat more dramatic of a falling out with her own father. The guy's a piece of shit parasite who totally fucked over his entire family while wearing a shit-eating grin the whole time. I think, watching that relationship dissolve in a thermo-nuclear family humanitarian catastrophe, I learned what a truly awful father looks like. And that's not what my dad looked like. He'd made mistakes, but as the rest of this book attests, I've made more than a few of my own volition. But he wasn't a bad guy. Actually, he's a really, really good guy. He's probably always been my best friend, and I'm just realizing it now. We've even gone for walks and gone over my (late) taxes at the time of this writing. He promised me something big: that I'll never go homeless, which is one of my greatest fears, as it essentially signals my end if I end up on the street. The next step is educating and meeting my sister and mother. I've offered the olive branch through my dad and psychiatrist. I pray it works. And I don't generally use that word. I need a family. My family.

FIFTY

2020

I'm in between two dates, Christmas, and the practising for Christmas dinner at my parents' house with my grandma, sister, brother-in-law, nephews, and Chuckles in attendance. We wanted to make sure we could sit down in peace without causing a ruckus. It went off without a hitch. I have Christmas presents picked out for my whole family, and I'm excited for my mom's legendary treacle pudding and my grandma's complementary baklava. I also have to watch out now, though, aging as only an overweight, sedentary, degenerate like me can: I have high cholesterol, blood pressure, and blood sugar. My blood is basically, literally, a cannabis-infused honey oil.

Reconnecting with my family came faster than any of us anticipated, and much more aggressively (in a good way). I was initially going to leapfrog from one family member to the next, with the assistance and presence of my psychiatrist, but the pandemic changed everything.

My grandfather isn't getting any better. If I want to be part of this process, I need to speed up the pace on my own healing so that I can establish some sort of meaningful reconciliation.

One day in early autumn we agreed to the terms: all superficial talk. That's it. Just keep it civil. Chuckles and I walked over to my parents' place, and we sat in the backyard and talked. I was totally sober. Not even a leaf. It was a perfect autumn day. Sunny but with enough chill to warrant pants and a sweater. I pointed at their firepit.

—Maybe some marshmallows?

"Maybe next time you come over. Maybe with the boys. Don't want the neighbours saying anything."

My dad just seemed gentle. This wasn't what I'd been remembering of life with my parents. I'd been clinging to bad memories. Prioritizing them. Amplifying them to the point of distortion. I'd been fostering hate on a diet of distorted styles of thinking. They weren't anything like that.

The full realization of how sick I'd been hit me. How sick I must have been. But I honoured my word and kept talking superficially.

We discussed politics (holy shit, a lot had happened), nature walks, old vacations. The deepest it really got was touching on memories of our dog Java, whom Dad was happy to finally show me his latest painting of. I'd forgotten what nice people they are. We agreed to do it again. And we did. And it worked. Occasionally the conversation might stray to something sensitive, but Chuckles is deft in her ability to deflect topics to safer terrains. We hung out with them a number of times. Dinner with the folks just became another way to spend a few nights a week. My dad's a great chef, and my mom's mounds of treacle pudding, covered in custard, portal me to positive childhood memories.

My sister was next. The obstacle was Christmas. We decided on that practice run. She, Chuckles, and I sat in my parents' backyard in the rain, under the patio umbrellas, with masks on. Chuckles did most of the talking and, as it turns out, gets along well with my sister, but she told me afterward that my sister had been looking at me the whole time. I hadn't been able to face her and consequently didn't notice. She did seem more forgiving than I'd remembered her, though. Like my dad, she was gentle. Maybe she was also exhausted and wanted her family back.

I never really felt like I *knew* my sister. She's a very elusive character. Growing up we largely treated each other like furniture … we got along fine and didn't give it much thought. But if you try to prod a little, you'll find that she's not so much a closed book as, like, a play … or just straight-up not a book. Chuckles had been intimidated by what we interpreted as my sister's aloofness but eventually mustered the courage to just ask:

"What goes through your mind when you pause for so long between when we say something and you answer?"

My sister predictably took a long time to formulate a response:

"I was just thinking how that tree looks like it has a face in it."

Ohhh, true. She's *my* sister. That makes sense.

I was worried, though, how my nephews must see me. The younger one probably wouldn't recall me at all, but the older one used to call me his "best big buddy," and when I parted ways from the family, he didn't get a personalized explanation. He thought he was, in some way, responsible. And that gutted me.

I had to do right by him. By all of them. Once I'd finally realized they bore me no real ill will, which is really what I'd expected from everyone (ever the optimist), and I reintroduced myself to my nephews, it was like nothing had ever happened. They were hopping all over me by the end of the night. The team was back together. Maybe it's magic, or maybe it's our British repression, but it's working.

* * *

My psychiatrist says I've been in remission for about a year now. I'm on a solid cocktail of psychiatric medication, along with pot. And that's it. I've washed my hands of it. All the other drugs. I don't want to go as deep as I've been anymore. Tickle the surface, maybe ... but I never want to break the meniscus of reality again. I never want to go free diving with chemically induced psychosis.

Something I *have* started using with the regularity of an addiction is spice. Capsaicin is amazing. I love insanely spicy peppers and hot sauces. Scotch bonnets, ghost peppers, California Reapers, Pepper X ... I go all the way up the ladder. I crave the feeling of having a tongue of molten glass. The intensity of the adrenalin rush. The alternating waves of hot and cold that come from the napalm-infused fruit. And spice always makes me smile. When I'm feeling down, I can reliably go to the fridge, grab some of the spiciest shit on the planet, and immediately break out in a sweaty smile. It elevates my mood. Not as much as, say, MDMA, but it does it in a cleaner, more reliable way, with no burnout.

But I do still wonder. Do I need these psychiatric compounds? These five interlacing molecules designed to keep me
in check? Would maybe something else do the trick? Would
eating magic mushrooms once in a while do basically the same
thing? Or more? I've had and seen great results with therapeutic
psychedelics, but having used them so long in a recreational context, even after knowing of their healing and spiritual
properties, I feel like I've perverted something that could have
been beautiful.

Maybe someday I'll come back to it. Under a doctor's supervision, I'd love to begin a microdosing regime. Pair that with
exercise and regular meditation. Yeah. And one day, once it's
legal, I'd like a whole psychotropic garden, a cove of poisons
Mithridates would be proud of. I want one day to have a green-
house with an aquaponic/vermiponic/bioponic set-up where I
grow all sorts of medicinal plants and spicy peppers and fungi
along the principles of companion planting, and raise a bal-
anced ecosystem of fish of all different sorts. It'll fit well in my
hippie commune.

I like the image of me as an old man, wandering through
the woods one spring with half a gram of *Psilocybe semilanceata*
in my stomach, searching for wild forest mushrooms like a Paul
Stamets/shaman hybrid, like my ancestors, and being all right
with that. I hope my mind can be all right with that. I hope the
world can be all right with that.

* * *

In early August I was out of money and desperate. I could, by
now, beg for money from my parents, having been folded back
into the family, but I wanted to do it myself. As always. I was

still depressed as all fuck, but I employed some opposite action, and I completed the certificate that would allow me to legally sell cannabis. Very crucial: having a criminal record bars you from working in the cannabis industry (which is stupid as fuck, but whatever) so I feel especially blessed to have so inelegantly danced my way around the repercussions of my actions.

First was the certificate. About sixty bucks and a few hours of online work. I noticed that some of their content was wrong ... but I played along and answered how they wanted me to. Chuckles tailored my resumé, and I began getting bites immediately. My combined background of banking, editing, and good ol' fashioned hustling was great bait. Working at The Mercy was the golden ticket. I had a few interviews, but most of the businesses seemed so in flux themselves: they weren't entirely sure what roles they were hiring for; they weren't sure when their store would be finished and ready to open; even in a few cases, they were still waiting for the final paperwork to register them as legal cannabis resellers.

Eventually I got an interview with a place that seemed to have its shit a bit more together. I was totally new to the legal cannabis industry. I'd only bought legal herb once, and I was disappointed by so much about it. I shone like moissanite in my interview. I was obviously much better informed about the fundamentals of the product than almost anyone else. I didn't know the brands, but I knew the science. On my way out the door the budtender manning the counter asked me if I was going to buy anything.

—I'll buy your weed when you pay me to sell it.

And now I'm back in my element, slingin' green. It's great!

It's still, ultimately, a retail job. You gotta deal with the people. And, like, 95 percent of people are, in my estimation, just not worth the effort. But I have to remember: it's not them I'm working for; it's their money.

You meet some interesting people, though, for sure. Old ladies with stories about tripping from Amsterdam to the Hindu Kush, on more than just weed. Or fresh-faced nineteen-year-olds buying legal pot for the first time and astounded at the array of interesting, novel manifestations of the herb. One interaction in mid-November, however, has had a longer lasting impact on me than I'd ever thought I would have selling weed, short of getting shot or something.

In mid-November this lady comes in to buy a joint. The interaction is nothing special, but I have a weird feeling that I recognize this lady from somewhere. At the end I punch in her order to my tablet and ask for her name (which I have altered for her privacy and entertainment):

"[Editer.]"

—No shit!

I recognize her from the writing world. I'm not sure if she remembers this, but I cornered her at one of her readings and spat some of my madcap poetry at her once. I pull down my mask to show my whole face.

"Oh shit! It's you!"

—Haha, yep, little old me. How are you doin'?

"I'm good! Just got a new job at [publishing house]! I'm excited about it. What about you? What are you up to?"

—I'm about to sell you a joint of a very relaxing strain of cannabis. That's pretty much what I've got going on these days.

"No, like, are you working on anything?"

In all honesty, I'd kind of given up on writing. At least for the moment. I'd always felt this compulsion to write my ideas: because the thoughts were just sooo precious they *had* to be shared. Thing was, the sorts of people I could share with were few and far between. As you may have noticed by now, my writing style is not likely conducive to being read by many members of the great unwashed. After writing hundreds of pages of prose and poetry and film scripts and essays, I just couldn't get anyone to read it. So fuck it. I'd keep the thoughts to myself and maybe stop alienating people, like a more self-involved Henry Darger who still harboured secret desires to be celebrated. Just be the simple, quiet guy with his own universe happening. I hadn't written in quite a while. It had been even longer since I'd submitted to a publisher, hating the process of jumping through hoops only to hear nothing back. Fuck haute couture and the Canadian glitterati.

—Yeah, I've got a poetry collection I'm ready to start shopping around, and I've got, like, a creative non-fiction sort of autobiographical novella-type thing. It's pretty fucked up, though, and I've been told there aren't many companies that might be interested. I tried to contact a company I was recommended by another writer, but the publisher said they were going out of business. Too niche.

"Can you describe it really roughly?"

—I guess it's kind of like a more heartfelt *Fear and Loathing in Las Vegas* ...

"Cool, well, my company is accepting submissions right now for non-fiction actually. You should submit."

—I fuckin' hate submissions.

"Everyone hates submissions. Just try it. You never know."

So I submitted it.

And about a month went by.

Then I saw a message from Editer in my inbox. It was December 23.

~Hey, can I call you tonight? What's your number?~

This was a much more personalized response than I've ever gotten from a publisher. Usually it's just radio silence. I responded with the requisite information and after about an hour my phone buzzed.

—Hello? [Editer]?

"Hey. Sorry for the wait. So, I read it. And, umm. I really liked it. And I'm gonna be presenting this to the team ... so it's not, like, a firm thing yet ... but I have a good feeling. I don't know about the poetry ... how we can work that ... we don't publish poetry ... and I don't wanna say you're getting a book yet. But ... you're probably getting a book."

HOLY FUCK.

—I'm really glad you smoke weed.

"OK. Don't get your hopes up too much. I'm gonna keep pushing from my end. Wish me luck!"

Fuck it. My hopes are up. Someone's going to read my book. People will read my thoughts. You are reading this, are you not?

I feel a sense of guilt, in a strange way. Guilt for the people who won't be published just because I will be. After all, what difference is there between me and them, other than that I had this miracle moment that pushed me to take this suggested chance? Sure, our writing is different, and our lives are different, and it's naive to believe that a publishing house would take a risk on someone they didn't believe in ... and I had to submit and go through a review process, too ... but what sort of irony is there in an intrinsically outsider artist securing one of the few coveted spots occupied by published authors, largely by means of a random interaction with a tenuously known peer (I was quite surprised Editer recognized me at all) ...

It really is all in who you know, innit?

This guilt, however, pales in comparison to another complex of feelings that pervades my every waking moment: fuck, all y'all, this is my life.

Ever since I was a kid, one of my greatest desires was to get other people to think like me. Or, at least, to understand the way I think and be able to act accordingly. Maybe that's why I proliferated so many psychedelics and indoctrinated so many future psychonauts. I'd spike the groundwater with LSD if I could. Maybe that's why I studied philosophy. I wanted to stop feeling alone. I wanted to connect to other people. And maybe that's why I started writing, which could possibly be an even more effective way of connecting with someone than selling them colourful bits of paper. Writing lasts.

This will all probably read like the demented little sibling of "Jabberwocky."

Nuts

```
The craziest thing is wishing
Interesting people will listen.

Shouldn't — but, I always figure
I'm special, like, I'll be bigger

Eventually. See, something must
Happen, or else I'll go cold, just

Ice — as in, "Hit me with one
On the rocks," and then done

With the fancy shit. Kafka
Stayed suckin' on Betrach-

Tung way longer than any
Piece of Bukowski's many
```

```
Whore-inspired, prosaic-feces
Masquerading as indecencies

He'd invented — like the new coliseum
Needed reruns of a pride in Te Deum.

But, maybe it does. I would be the ass
Hole full of spunk, guts, and Levinas

Extract from the exodus of ecstasy-
Era, Boom-Echo, debts-and-dream

Addled consciousness, or conscience
My folks call "a future" [sic: options]

Who'd suggest it. Sick: a word no worse
For the wearer of perspective than
     "Verse"

Holds in its pit of obsessive pursuit
After little perfections wear through …

So, let's all swing round for round
Is where this poem's going, drowned

In dialectic with solipsists —
Another anonymous monolith.
```

So I guess that's how this ends. Nowhere and full of promise. I never really got to a lot of the stories. I could go on for a while, but my memory isn't so good. I always figured I'd write my first book of poetry, have it out in my early twenties (I was a bit cocksure), then die from either a drug overdose or some other form of misadventure. Now I'm in my early thirties and my first book is a memoir, and Chuckles Skullfucker and I have plans for after this. I want to lead a life. I want to lead a good life.

I just hope none of this shit hangs over my head.

Acknowledgements

Thank you to Julie Mannell for catching my falling star. Thank you to Charleen Sye for making my wishes come true. Thanks to you, your thoughts and perspectives, for seeing my vision and sharing it.

Thanks to my family, both those of blood and belief: those who are here with me, those who have been, and those who are yet to be. You drive me. I know I'm not an easy person to know too closely. I love you.

Thanks are in order for the whole Dundurn Press team. Thank you to every person who laboured over my typos and imaginary words; thank you to every person who worked on the marketing, accounting, decision making ... just everything. Thank you. Thank you to Laura Boyle and anyone else associated with the design for this cover. It's so fucking appropriate.

Thank you, also, to whoever may be reading this right now. You. Yeah, thank You. Whether you like it or not, I exist in your mind, and I would like to acknowledge the space for my story that you are providing.

Now, I would like to recognize the inspiration that the Janus of mental health/illness has provided me. It continues to inspire me. My experience and yours alike. Thank you to everyone who knows what that means. You are my kin.

Thank you. Thank you. Thank you.

— Yours

About the Author

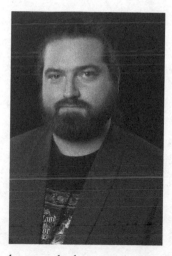 Born in Toronto to Canadian parents, Andrew Brobyn was raised overseas, following his father's career, first to Barbados and then the Channel Islands to Jersey. Upon returning to Toronto with a fusion accent of aristocratic British with a Bajan inflection, he soon learned it would be hard to coalesce with Canadianism.

Over the course of his adolescence he began experimenting with a number of substances, for a number of reasons: to fit in, to push the limit, to see trippy stuff scrawled on the walls, but most intensely, to unfold the fabrics the world is woven of. For better or worse.

Andrew now works in the legal cannabis market, pursuing his artistic passions of writing and creating nefariously dark cartoons whenever time permits.